Protecting Your Health Privacy

Protecting Your Health Privacy

A Citizen's Guide to Safeguarding the Security of Your Medical Information

Jacqueline Klosek

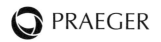

PRAEGER

AN IMPRINT OF ABC-CLIO, LLC
Santa Barbara, California • Denver, Colorado • Oxford, England

Library of Congress Cataloging-in-Publication Data

Klosek, Jacqueline, 1972–
    Protecting your health privacy : a citizen's guide to safeguarding the security of your
medical information / Jacqueline Klosek.
        p. cm.
    Includes bibliographical references and index.
    ISBN 978-0-313-38717-3 (hard copy : alk. paper)—ISBN 978-0-313-38718-0 (ebook)
1. Medical records—Access control. 2. Privacy, Right of. 3. Data protection. I. Title.

R864.K56   2011
651.5'04261—dc22   2010034862

ISBN: 978-0-313-38717-3
EISBN: 978-0-313-38718-0

15   14   13   12   11   1   2   3   4   5

This book is also available on the World Wide Web as an eBook.
Visit www.abc-clio.com for details.

Praeger
An Imprint of ABC-CLIO, LLC

ABC-CLIO, LLC
130 Cremona Drive, P.O. Box 1911
Santa Barbara, California 93116-1911

This book is printed on acid-free paper ∞

Manufactured in the United States of America

Protecting Your Health Privacy *is dedicated to my beloved Labrador, Brian, an eternal optimist, a great running partner, and an all-around best friend, and to my brother, Jason Klosek, a true inspiration and fabulous human being.*

Contents

Author's Note

I became interested in privacy many years ago when I was working in the Brussels office of Deloitte LLC as a legal advisor. At that time, comprehensive privacy legislation (Directive EC 95/46) with extraterritorial reach was entering into force in Europe, and many enterprises throughout the world were concerned with compliance. As one of only a few Americans on a team that was providing advice to U.S. corporations seeking to do business in Europe and encountering difficulties in complying with the European privacy laws, a significant part of my duties involved advising American companies on European privacy requirements. Spending a lot of time working in this area, my interest in the topic grew, and I eventually wrote my first book, *Data Privacy in the Information Age*, about the differences between American and European approaches to privacy.

Since then, I have remained involved in and focused upon privacy on a professional and personal level. My interest level in medical privacy in particular ratcheted up after I was asked to teach a seminar on HIPAA at Seton Hall University Law School. Discussing and debating the issues with smart, motivated, and energetic students helped me to look at some of the issues in a new light, while also fostering greater interest in the topic.

My interests in medical privacy were also impacted by personal issues. Like most people, I have had my share of health challenges, from having cardiac surgery as a toddler to being diagnosed with Crohn's disease in my twenties. Fortunately, I have been able to embrace my health challenges and convert them into fuel to help me grow stronger mentally and physically. Thus, I am rather open about what I have faced and what I have done, mainly so that I may be able to share with others information about things that have helped me in the hope that it may also help them.

At the same time as I can see how openness about my health challenges was the right way for me, I can also appreciate that, for a myriad of reasons, others facing various health challenges may not be as able or as willing to disclose what they are going through. And I feel wholeheartedly that they should have that right to keep their privacy. In the immediate aftermath of a shocking diagnosis, even the strongest and most open people will need time to adjust and accept the diagnosis and they should be allowed to do so in private. In fact, I am not advocating for broad personal disclosure of one's health challenges. As will be shown in this book, the disclosure of medical information can have significant implications on one's employment, finances, and relationships. The point is that it is a personal choice, and every person should be entitled to make that choice for him- or herself.

As will be discussed throughout this book, doctor-patient confidentiality is a fundamental tenet of health care that can be traced back to ancient times. Today, however, many constituencies beyond health care providers have access to and/or interest in individuals' health care information. This makes protecting the privacy of health information far more of a challenge than it had been in the immediate past.

I wrote this book not only to inform individuals about the laws that are in place to protect their health privacy and to discuss the limitations of those laws, but also to inform people about the actions that they may be taking to compromise their own medical privacy and empower them with the tools needed to better protect themselves against unwanted intrusions into their health privacy.

Acknowledgments

First, on a personal note, I am grateful to many people who have supported and guided me along the way. Much appreciation is owed to my dad, John, who read all of my drafts and always offered constructive feedback. His text messages, admittedly brief and most likely sent from his boat or hammock, showed me that he actually read my drafts and helped to motivate me toward the finish line. I must also thank my mother, my aunt Mare, and my brothers, Michael and Jason. While their feedback on my drafts may be a bit overdue, they are always there to cheer me on and encourage me. I would be remiss if I failed to express my deep appreciation to Tom Lozinski. Although Tom sometimes discouraged me from continued writing, suggesting surfing, rock climbing, and biking as plausible alternatives, he was always available for guidance when I needed it. He is a very informed person who I have learned to count on for interesting discussions and debates. He provokes me and challenges me so that I am better able to question my assumptions and see the other side of an issue, and he kept me happy and grounded throughout this process. In that regard, gratitude is also owed to Tom's mom, Roseann Lozinski, who not only offered support and encouragement to me, but who also gave so much of her time in reviewing and editing my manuscript. Finally, I wish to acknowledge my nephews Mathew and William and my niece Meredith, just for being so cute, fun, and full of life and energy. My wish for you little cherubs is that you never need any of the advice in this book. Stay well and be happy.

I must also acknowledge those whose valuable assistance contributing to this book. In particular, I wish to thank Lawrence Adler, Gabriel Bouskila, and Jon Whiten for their expert research skills and assistance. I must also thank them for maintaining positive, happy attitudes throughout the process and going with the flow, even though I must have tested their patience on at least a few occasions. Larry and Gabe, as you complete your respective journeys through law school, know that I have every confidence of your future success. I am also grateful to my editors, Robert Hutchinson and Valentina Tursini for having confidence in me, supporting my efforts, and providing great advice.

Legal notice: This book reflects my own views and opinions and is based upon research into sources believed to be accurate. It is not an official opinion of my employer, Goodwin Procter LLP. This book is not legal advice. Neither the publisher nor the author assume any liability for any errors or omissions, or for how this book or its contents are used or interpreted, or for any consequences resulting directly or indirectly from the use of this book. For legal, financial, medical, strategic, or any other type of advice, please personally consult the appropriate professional.

Introduction

Whatever I see or hear in the lives of my patients, whether in connection with my professional practice or not, which ought not to be spoken of outside, I will keep secret, as considering all such things to be private.

So long as I maintain this Oath faithfully and without corruption, may it be granted to me to partake of life fully and the practice of my art, gaining the respect of all men for all time. However, should I transgress this Oath and violate it, may the opposite be my fate.[1]

UNDERSTANDING HEALTH PRIVACY

Privacy is a sacred value to Americans. The right to privacy, while not set out explicitly in our Constitution, is well established in our legal system and is a tenet of our common law. In addition, as will be discussed throughout this book, lawmakers have enacted a number of laws and regulations to provide protection to various aspects of privacy. Among all aspects of private life that individuals seek to protect as confidential, heath is often a leading issue. For many people, information about health and medical status is among the most private and sensitive information.

Although privacy is a well-established part of our legal system, it is a complex concept that is not easily defined. In fact, the proper definition of privacy is something that has been the subject of very intense debate by a vast number of scholars, attorneys, and other experts. While there has not been universal agreement on the meaning of privacy, many different working definitions have been proposed.

In the seminal U.S. Supreme Court case, *Olmstead v. United States*, Justice Louis Brandeis characterized privacy as "the right to be let alone."[2] In the modern age, privacy sometimes focuses on specific rights, such as the right to be free from unwanted marketing, from invasive searches, or from intrusive surveillance—whether by government or by private interests, such as corporations. Concepts of privacy are also contextual, and the idea—as experienced on a personal level—may mean different things to different people or in different situations.[3]

In the domain of health information, privacy often encompasses not only privacy, but also confidentiality and security. While the proper and complete definition of privacy can be debated at length (and will likely continue to be debated), it generally concerns the collection, storage, and usage of information that identifies a particular individual. While the terms "privacy" and "confidentiality" are sometimes used interchangeably, there are subtle distinctions that are worthy of mention. Confidentiality typically concerns how information that is gathered is best protected. For example, confidentiality prevents physicians from disclosing information shared with them by a patient. Meanwhile, privacy often deals with access to, rather than disclosure of, information. Security helps ensure privacy by protecting health records from unauthorized access and use.

The Importance of Health Privacy

There are numerous important reasons for placing a high value on protecting the privacy, confidentiality, and security of health information. After all, medical records can include some of the most intimate details about a person's life, the most sensitive information that people often want protected. In addition to documenting a patient's physical and mental health, medical records can include details on a patient's social behaviors, personal relationships, and financial status.[4] Accordingly, there can be tangible consequences to the unauthorized use or disclosure of medical information. When personally identifiable health information, for example, is disclosed to third parties outside of the doctor-patient relationship (such as an employer, an insurer, or even a friend or family member), it can result in various negative consequences, including stigma, embarrassment, or discrimination. Despite laws prohibiting discrimination, individuals suffering from certain ailments are often subject to prejudgment and discrimination. This is particularly the case when it comes to mental health problems, addictions, and other socially stigmatized diseases discussed later in this book, but it also applies to a host of other ailments. Unauthorized disclosures of health information can also result in more subtle effects, such as unwanted coddling, sympathy, and lowered expectations of the individual's abilities. All too often, once an individual is known to be suffering from a particular ailment, it impacts how people perceive and treat the person.

Surveys have shown that individuals are concerned about insurers and employers accessing their health information without their permission.[5] Such concerns are motivated largely by fear of possible discrimination, such as limits on job opportunities. Unfortunately, such fears may not always be so far-fetched. With the costs of health care continuing to rise, and with employers bearing a large portion of those costs, employers may be tempted to take health conditions into account when hiring employees. In fact, there have already been reports of retail giant Walmart basing some of its hiring decisions on the health of applicants.[6] As will be discussed in this book, federal and state laws place limits on the kinds of health-related inquiries employers can make of employees and prospective employees, but these protections are not bulletproof.

The importance of privacy goes well beyond a need to prevent embarrassment, discrimination, or identity theft. Ensuring privacy can promote more effective communication between physician and patient, which is essential for quality of care. Without some assurance of privacy, people may be reluctant to candidly and completely disclose sensitive information, even to their personal physicians. In this context, privacy and security can literally save lives. People who do not believe their information will be kept private may delay seeking—or not seek at all—life-enhancing and life-saving treatments. This is particularly the case with respect to certain illnesses that are socially stigmatized. Patients suffering from certain ailments, such as the socially stigmatizing diseases examined in Chapter 7, may avoid or delay treatment until they can pay in cash in order to avoid the creation of a paper trail with their insurer.

Ensuring the confidentiality of adolescents and teenagers' medical information is especially important, particularly when the issue involves potential trouble with the law or with family. Researchers have found that when adolescents believe that health services are not confidential, they will be less likely to seek care, particularly for medical concerns involving substance abuse and reproductive health.[7] Other researchers have found the same result with adult populations, finding that the willingness of individuals to make disclosures necessary to aid mental health and substance abuse treatment may decrease as the perceptions of a breach of confidentiality increase.[8] There are similar concerns with respect to serious, transmittable disease, such as HIV/AIDS. The Centers for Disease Control (CDC) has estimated that an astonishing 300,000 personals living with HIV infection are unaware of their status.[9] With the stigma associated with HIV/AIDS, unless people can be sure that their privacy and confidentiality will be maintained, they may be less likely to get tested and seek treatment.

In order for people to seek help with serious ailments about problems that may affect not only themselves, but also their families, communities, and society at large, they need to feel secure that their privacy will be protected.

Some experts have depicted privacy as a basic human right, with intrinsic value of its own.[10] This view of privacy is consistent with major international human rights conventions, treaties, and other instruments that identify privacy as a fundamental human right.[11] Adherents to this view might advocate for health privacy rights on the basis that as human beings, we have an intrinsic right to the protection of our private health lives.

Individual Expectations of Health Privacy

The biggest step toward protecting health privacy in this era was the creation of Health Insurance Portability and Accountability Act (HIPAA).[12] This federal legislation, which was passed by Congress in 1995, was created in part to help keep patients' electronic health records private. But surveys and other research consistently show that, while individuals value health privacy, they are concerned about the efficacy of this and other current protections. For example, a 2005 survey conducted by Forrester Research found that 67 percent of respondents remained concerned about the privacy of their medical records—despite the federal protections under HIPAA. The survey also revealed that the majority of people were "largely unaware" of their medical privacy rights. More specifically, only 59 percent of respondents reported a recollection of receiving a HIPAA privacy notice from their health care provider. Further, a surprising number of respondents—27 percent—believed that they had more rights than HIPAA actually guaranteed.[13] Two years later, a poll by United Press International and Zogby International found that more than half the 10,258 U.S. participants expressed privacy concerns regarding their medical records and information, with African Americans and Hispanics having greater concerns over the issue than Caucasians.[14] Even more recently, the Harris Poll in 2008 reported that a surprising percentage of people are skeptical about the ability of doctors to keep their information private. The poll showed that 69 percent of people asked had either heard or read about medical records being lost or stolen from doctors' offices, clinics, hospitals, and other medical facilities. The poll observed that "[f]or over two-thirds of the general public to recall hearing about medical data breaches is a very high topic awareness figure."[15] These figures provide an insight as to what the public thinks of the medical industry's ability to keep its information private, and it does not bode well for doctors, hospitals, and other health care providers. Such concerns are likely to grow as the government works to encourage more widespread use of electronic health records.[16]

THREATS TO HEALTH PRIVACY

While patient confidentiality is a very well established tenet of medical care, the task of securing the privacy and confidentiality of health information has become increasingly complex in recent years for a number of reasons. One of these is technology. While technology is essential to protecting data, the use of technology to transmit, share, and store personal information aids in the proliferation of such information, thereby also contributing to the security risks of that information. Consider, for example, some recent well-publicized reports of cases in which the privacy and security of medical records have been compromised:

- Health care workers have lost laptops and other portable devices containing patients' unencrypted medical information.
- Paper documents containing medical data were found blowing around in the street after being placed in a recycling bin for pickup.
- Medical providers faxed medical records to the incorrect recipient.
- Pharmacies tossed hard copies of prescription records in dumpsters without first shredding the papers.
- Medical workers have accessed records of patients out of curiosity or for profit, and without medical cause or proper authorization.
- An insurance company published a patient's actual medical records in an employee training manual.

With the enactment of laws requiring notification of breaches involving medical information, public reports of these kinds are likely to continue and may in fact worsen. This is not to say that breaches were not occurring before, but now that there are laws that require entities suffering from certain breaches to make individual or public announcements of the breach, we may see more breaches in the headlines.

One of the biggest threats to medical privacy is simple human error, often resulting in lost information, inadvertent release of information, misclassification of information, improper disclosure, and other types of data misuse. The news is replete with stories of lost or stolen laptops that led to the breach of large amounts of medical information. Chapter 3, "Data Insecurity, Breaches, and ID Theft," will explore in greater detail how inadequate data security and human error can result in data breaches, misappropriation of information, and, in some cases, even identity theft and other harm.

While advances in information technology can improve information security, increased computerization and digitization also poses threats to the privacy and security of medical information. Password-protected files, encryption, and computers may enhance privacy and security. However, digitization also facilitates the storage of massive amounts of data in minute spaces, which can make data more vulnerable. For example, an intruder walking off with an unencrypted laptop—or an even smaller portable device like a flash drive—can steal information about a tremendous number of individuals. Risks also arise out of the increasing use of networks and cloud computing. Information housed on a network is accessible from anywhere at any time, which means a larger number of people might be able to access it. This, in turn, increases the possibility of errors, misuse of information, and data breaches.

A number of third parties also have access to medical information, further threatening individual health privacy. For example, insurance companies may access and review medical records prior to extending coverage or approving certain treatments. Pharmaceutical companies may also have access to certain medical information.

Legal processes, including court subpoenas, can also threaten medical privacy. Often, individuals are not even aware when their medical records have been subpoenaed, as the subpoena is issued to the party controlling the information, such as the health insurance company, health care provider, or even a technology company providing services to one of those entities. Of potentially greater concern, sometimes the recipient of the subpoena may not adequately screen the records and may mistakenly release private medical information that is not actually being subpoenaed.

Our medical system is in the midst of an important transformation that may impact the privacy and security of our medical information. Under the stimulus legislation, the government is to direct $45 billion to launch a national shift to electronic records. Individual doctors are to be given as much as $44,000 to spend on digitizing health records.[17] The incentives seem quite likely to motivate providers to make the transition to electronic records. Given where we are at the present and where we are to be in a relatively short period of time, the changes are to be quick and vast. At the present, less than one in five of the country's 600,000 doctors and 5,000 hospitals now use electronic medical records, but by 2015, all are supposed to be maintaining medical records electronically.[18]

There is a diversity of opinions about what the transition of electronic health records will mean to the privacy and security of medical information.[19] Many experts point out that electronic medical records do entail risks, not only to the privacy and security of a patient's privacy, but also to his or her health.[20] Other thought leaders in this field have pointed to evidence that shows that the increased use of electronic technology can lead to reduced medical errors.[21] The potential risks and benefits of the increased use of electronic technology in medical care will be discussed further throughout this book.

OVERVIEW OF THE LEGAL LANDSCAPE

As mentioned previously, HIPAA is the key health privacy legislation in the United States. Accordingly, a substantial portion of this book will be devoted to examining the individual rights that HIPAA conveys upon patients and the obligations that it imposes on health care providers and other "covered entities," such as health insurance providers and health care clearing houses (each a covered entity).

HIPAA's Privacy Rule and Security Rule defines and limits the circumstances in which an individual's protected heath information (PHI) may be used or disclosed by covered entities. Generally, a covered entity may not use or disclose PHI, except either (1) as the privacy rule permits or requires, or (2) as the individual who is the subject of the information (or the individual's personal representative) authorizes in writing. The privacy rule also conveys additional rights on individuals, such as the right to obtain copies of records containing PHI and to request an accounting of all disclosures of records containing PHI. In addition, the rule imposes a number of duties and obligations on covered entities. For example, covered entities must designate an individual who oversees the organization's compliance efforts. They must also conduct training of their workforce. HIPAA also establishes technical, administrative, and organizational specifications that covered entities must comply with in order to protect peoples' personal health information.

Health information privacy and security is currently undergoing significant changes. To further encourage the transition to electronic health records, the Obama administration has recognized the need to further enhance the privacy and security of medical records. As a result, when legislators enacted the American Reinvestment and Recovery Act of 2009 (ARRA),[22] the federal stimulus package, they included the Health Information Technology for Economic and Clinical Health Act, or HITECH Act,[23] which is ushering in significant changes to the regulation of health privacy. This book will include a detailed discussion of the provisions and likely impact of the HITECH Act.

States also play an important role in the protection of health privacy. While HIPAA and HITECH have established a basic floor for privacy protection on a national level, they have not gone far enough. For instance, enforcement of HIPAA is lacking and it does not allow people to bring individual lawsuits. States can enact legislation that provides greater protection than the federal legislation. This book will examine the role that certain states are playing in the protection of health privacy.

THE PURPOSE AND ORGANIZATION OF THIS BOOK

This is an opportune time to examine health privacy as, going forward, these issues will likely become even more complex. Recent changes in law and technology will have a dramatic impact on the privacy, security, and control of individuals' health information and, ultimately, the direction of their health care. People must be aware of the current legal framework so they can be empowered to protect themselves and their families. While presenting detailed information about health privacy and security law, this text will also analyze common practices of companies involved in the collection, use, and exchange of health information (such as health care providers, insurers, employers, social networking sites, and marketers). Particular attention will be devoted to the evolving world of personal health records, the potential impact of reform efforts, and the special issues faced by people dealing with substance addiction, mental health challenges, and other socially stigmatized diseases.

Chapter 1, "Understanding Health Privacy Law," introduces the current legal framework applicable to medical privacy. While a substantial portion of this chapter will be devoted to HIPAA, the chapter will also explore other federal and state laws that play a role in the privacy of human health. The chapter will explore how these laws protect privacy, as well as the limitations of the existing legal framework.

Chapter 2, "Your Rights under HIPAA and How to Exercise Them," informs about the scope of privacy rights and how those rights may be exercised. While current laws to protect the privacy and security of health information are in many ways insufficient, they do convey certain important individual rights, including the right to receive notice of a covered entity's privacy practices, the right to access medical records, the right to be notified about when and with whom a covered entity shares your medical records, and the right to control certain uses and disclosures of medical information.

Chapter 3, "Data Insecurity, Breaches, and ID Theft," examines the serious and growing problem of data insecurity. Without effective security, there can be no privacy. Individuals whose health information has been breached may face harm in the form of loss of insurance, discrimination, or identity theft. In addition to examining the problem of data insecurity and the consequences of breaches, this chapter will provide advice on how to best protect against data breach.

Chapter 4, "Taking It in Your Own Hands: Personal Health Records," explores the new realm of personal health records (PHRs). While PHRs can allow for greater control of one's own medical information, PHR vendors are not regulated in the same way that covered entities are. Patients will have to do a lot of legwork to understand the practices and policies of the PHR vendors, prior to sharing their sensitive medical information with these entities. This chapter will offer some tips and recommendations on selecting a PHR vendor and ensuring that your information is protected when stored in a PHR.

In Chapter 5, "Your Health Privacy at Work," our discussion moves to the workplace. Health privacy at work is a crucial issue. Many of the legal protections under HIPAA will not protect employees, even though there are many risks to health privacy in the workplace. This chapter will explore the diverse selection of health privacy issues that impact employees, including discussions of wellness centers at work, hiring and screening processes, social networking and employers, insurance, and genetic testing.

Chapter 6, "Marketing Your Health," examines how companies might be using your medical information for various marketing purposes. There is a wide range of activities that can fall under the general umbrella of marketing. In some instances, an entity may use your medical information to market related products and services to you. In other cases, an entity may sell your information to other companies so that they may market products and services to you. Still, in other cases, companies may evaluate aggregated health information to analyze and understand trends and then sell or license the results of this data analysis to various third parties.

Chapter 7, "The Special Cases of Mental Health, Addiction, Socially Stigmatizing Diseases, and Other Intensely Private Health Matters," looks at special issues associated with mental health, addiction and substance abuse, and socially stigmatized diseases. While HIPAA is quite comprehensive, there are other laws, particularly at the state level, but at the federal level as well, that provide different or enhanced protections for this type of information.

Next, in Chapter 8, "International Perspectives in Health Privacy," we examine key privacy laws in place in several other countries. With health care reform being a very hot issue in the United States, it is particularly useful to evaluate how other countries that have more centralized systems of heath care protect the privacy and security of health information. Additionally, the countries that will be examined in this chapter have all elected to protect privacy through omnibus legislation that protects privacy regardless of what entities are collecting it and what industries are involved. This contrasts sharply with the approach of the United States, where privacy laws have been based upon particular industries and sectors of the economy. It is anticipated that reviewing the laws in place in these other jurisdictions might help in the assessment of the sufficiency of our sector-based approach.

Finally, the conclusion aims to provide further guidance on how individuals can take appropriate steps to protect their own health privacy. This final chapter aims to provide useful tools and checklists for those who may find it prudent to assume a greater role in the protection of their own medical privacy. The conclusion also offers suggestions on how we may wish to strengthen and/or otherwise modify existing legal protections applicable to the privacy and security of health information.

1

Understanding Health Privacy Laws

A BRIEF HISTORY OF HEALTH PRIVACY IN THE UNITED STATES

Protecting the privacy of medical information has been an important part of health care since at least 400 BCE, when the Hippocratic Oath declared: "What I may see or hear in the course of the treatment or even outside of the treatment in regard to the life of men, which on no account one must spread abroad, I will keep to myself, holding such things shameful to be spoken about."[1] This privacy pledge has been included in nearly all health care professionals' codes of ethics in the United States. The concept of confidentiality is engrained into the profession of medical practice, and most medical professionals hold the duty to maintain patient privacy as sacrosanct. For example, the first code of ethics of the American Medical Association, adopted in 1847, included the concept of confidentiality.[2]

Today, the Health Insurance Portability and Accountability Act of 1996 (HIPAA)[3] plays a significant role in the regulation of medical privacy. In fact, many people associate the very idea of health privacy with HIPAA. Nonetheless, medical privacy was legally protected long before HIPAA, a relatively recent law, was enacted. Prior to HIPAA, health privacy was protected primarily under a combination of federal and state constitutional law, as well as state common law and statutory protections. For example, prior to HIPAA, states had their own laws regarding the privacy and security of health information. Some were comprehensive, while others were specific to a type of ailment, such as HIV/AIDS or drug addiction.

The origins of many of these statutory and regulatory protections of privacy can be traced back to a 1973 report of an advisory committee to the U.S. Department of Health, Education and Welfare (HEW).[4] The report was designed to "call attention to issues of recordkeeping practice in the computer age that may have profound significance for us all" and to "provide a basis for establishing procedures that assure the individual a right to participate in a meaningful way in decisions about what goes into records about him and how that information shall be used."[5] In addition to giving individuals the right to control the collection, use, and disclosure of their information, the fair information practices outlined in the report also held those who collect that information responsible for safeguarding it.

The HEW report recognized the importance of protecting the privacy and security of personal information, recommending that:

- There must be no personal-data record-keeping systems whose very existence is secret.
- There must be a way for an individual to find out what information about him is in a record and how it is used.
- There must be a way for an individual to prevent information about him that is obtained for one purpose from being used or made available for other purposes without his consent.
- There must be a way for an individual to correct or amend a record of identifiable information about him.
- Any organization creating, maintaining, using, or disseminating records of identifiable personal data must assure the reliability of the data for their intended use and must take reasonable precautions to prevent misuse of the data.[6]

Subsequent to the HEW Report, in 1980, the Organization for Economic Cooperation and Development (OECD) built upon the core HEW fair information principles and created a set of eight fair information practices codified in the *OECD Guidelines on the Protection of Privacy and Transborder Flows of Personal Data* (OECD Guidelines).[7] These principles, which were agreed upon by OECD member countries, including the United States, form the basis of many modern privacy laws. Although they cover privacy generally and thus are not focused specifically on medical privacy, the OECD guidelines are worth mentioning given their influence on the development of privacy rights worldwide. Interestingly, the OECD guidelines are quite comprehensive, addressing a number of aspects of privacy protection, including security of information, accountability for privacy violations, obligations to ensure that information remains correct and up-to-date, and other key issues. The OECD guidelines are set forth in Table 1.1.

Although medical professionals have a long history of recognizing the importance of patient confidentiality and striving to protect it, over the years the privacy and security of personal health information have become increasingly vulnerable to a number of threats. Over time, as the delivery of health care has changed and technology has advanced, the number and type of individuals and organizations accessing individual health information has greatly expanded. In the not-too-distant past, one may have been able to see a local doctor about a medical problem and paid in full with cash for the medical care. In this context, it is likely that the doctor may have made handwritten

TABLE 1.1
OECD Guidelines on the Protection of Privacy and Transborder Flows of Personal Data

The Eight Fair Information Practices

1. **Collection Limitation Principle**. There should be limits to the collection of personal data, and any such data should be obtained by lawful and fair means and, where appropriate, with the knowledge or consent of the data subject.

2. **Data Quality Principle**. Personal data should be relevant to the purposes for which they are to be used, and, to the extent necessary for those purposes, should be accurate, complete, and kept up-to-date.

3. **Purpose Specification Principle**. The purposes for which personal data are collected should be specified not later than at the time of data collection and the subsequent use limited to the fulfillment of those purposes or such others as are not incompatible with those purposes and as are specified on each occasion of change of purpose.

4. **Use Limitation Principle**. Personal data should not be disclosed, made available, or otherwise used for purposes other than those specified in accordance with Paragraph 9 except: a) with the consent of the data subject; or b) by the authority of law.

5. **Security Safeguards Principle**. Personal data should be protected by reasonable security safeguards against such risks as loss or unauthorized access, destruction, use, modification, or disclosure of data.

6. **Openness Principle**. There should be a general policy of openness about developments, practices, and policies with respect to personal data. Means should be readily available of establishing the existence and nature of personal data, and the main purposes of their use, as well as the identity and usual residence of the data controller.

7. **Individual Participation Principle**. An individual should have the right:
   a) To obtain from a data controller, or otherwise, confirmation of whether or not the data controller has data relating to him;
   b) To have communicated to him data relating to him within a reasonable time; at a charge, if any, that is not excessive; in a reasonable manner; and in a form that is readily intelligible to him;
   c) To be given reasons if a request made under subparagraphs (a) and (b) is denied, and to be able to challenge such denial; and
   d) To challenge data relating to him and, if the challenge is successful, to have the data erased, rectified, completed, or amended.

8. **Accountability Principle**. A data controller should be accountable for complying with measures that give effect to the principles stated above.

notes about the patient and the care delivered, and those handwritten notes would have probably remained stored in a file cabinet in that doctor's office. Today, however, in most cases, access to individual health information is no longer limited to medical professionals who have the direct relationship with the patient subject to medical ethics codes. Rather, insurance companies, employers, government agencies, health-related Web sites, researchers, data aggregators, and potentially many others are now also privy to such information. Often these other parties are related to different, and in some cases, less stringent legal obligations with respect to data privacy and security.

HIPAA

Understanding HIPAA

Concerns about the increase in the numbers of individuals and entities that can have access to our medical information and the growth of potential threats to the privacy and security of that information have prompted the enactment of HIPAA, the first comprehensive federal law aimed at protecting the privacy and security of health information regulation.

Although HIPAA is commonly associated with privacy, that was not the main focus of the legislation. When HIPAA was first enacted, its initial impact was through its "portability" provisions, which make it easier for employees to continue their health insurance coverage when they lose their jobs or change employers. These portability provisions comprise the core of HIPAA. There is, however, a part of HIPAA, labeled "administrative simplification," that addresses the privacy and security of health information and establishes standards for certain electronic transactions.

The HIPAA Privacy Rule

The HIPAA Privacy Rule,[8] which became effective in April 2003, covers "protected health information" (hereinafter, PHI or protected health information) broadly defined as individually identifiable health information related to the past, present, or future physical or mental health or condition, the provision of health care to an individual, or the past, present, or future payment for the provision of health care to an individual.[9] While the HIPAA Privacy Rule applies to a broad class of information, it applies only to the extent that such information that is maintained by health care providers, health plans, and health clearinghouses (collectively known as covered entities) and, to a certain extent, their service providers, called business associates. While other entities, such as, for example, your health club, may have access to certain of your medical information, if the entity is not a covered entity or a business associate, that organization remains outside the scope of the HIPAA Privacy Rule.

The HIPAA Privacy Rule protects health privacy in a number of different ways: providing for certain individual rights, imposing restrictions on the use and disclosure of PHI, and requiring covered entities to implement administrative and procedural safeguards to ensure the privacy of PHI. In addition, the HIPAA Security Rule establishes a number of requirements that covered entities must follow to protect the security of PHI. Table 1.2 presents a high-level summary of the basic provisions of the HIPAA Privacy Rule.

TABLE 1.2
Summary of the HIPAA Privacy Rule

Establishes requirements for notice and acknowledgment:

- Health providers and certain health plans must provide a notice of privacy practices.
- Health providers are required to obtain an acknowledgment from individuals that they received the notice of privacy practices.

Establishes an individual's right to:

- Opt out of the facility directory (a directory used to store a patient's information, such as their name, condition, religious affiliation, etc.) or to request restrictions on other uses of PHI.
- Ask that communications be sent by alternative means or to an alternate address (for example, that correspondence be sent by e-mail or to a post office box).
- Access health information. It also establishes the limited situations wherein access may be denied.
- Request amendment of PHI.
- Obtain an accounting of disclosures of his or her PHI.

Establishes requirements for use and disclosure:

- Identifies uses and disclosures for which an authorization is required.
- Specifies who may authorize disclosure on behalf of an individual.
- Provides special protections for psychotherapy notes.
- Establishes a standard to limit the amount of information used or disclosed to the "minimum necessary" to accomplish the intended purpose.
- Requires that the covered entity identify members or classes of persons within its workforce who need access to PHI, the categories of information to which access is needed, and the conditions appropriate to such access.
- Establishes limitations on the use of PHI for fund-raising and procedures wherein individuals must be allowed to opt out.
- Establishes requirements for de-identification of health information that can be disclosed without authorization.

(Continued)

TABLE 1.2 (*Continued*)

Establishes certain administrative requirements:

- Requires that the covered entity designate a privacy official.
- Requires that the covered entity designate a contact person who can provide additional information and receive complaints.
- Requires that the covered entity train all members of its workforce on policies and procedures with respect to PHI.
- Requires that covered entities establish appropriate administrative, technical, and physical safeguards to protect health information.
- Establishes content or documentation requirements for policies and procedures, notices, authorizations, amendments, accounting of disclosures, complaints, and compliance.
- Addresses fees that may be charged for disclosure.

Preempts state law that is contrary to the privacy rule except when one of the following three conditions is met:

- An exception is made by the secretary of HHS.
- A provision in state law is more stringent than the privacy rule.
- The state law relates to public health surveillance and reporting.
- The state law relates to reporting for the purpose of management or financial audits, program monitoring and evaluation, and licensure or certification of facilities or individuals.

Individual Rights

The HIPAA Privacy Rule establishes a number of important individual rights. Specifically, the HIPAA Privacy Rule provides individuals with the right to receive a covered entity's notice of privacy practices. The notice is required to do several things:

- Describe the ways in which the covered entity may use and disclose protected health information.
- State the covered entity's duties to: (i) protect privacy of PHI, (ii) provide notice of privacy practices, and (iii) abide by the terms of the current notice.
- Describe an individual's rights, including the right to complain to the U.S. Department of Health and Human Services (HHS) and to the covered entity if they believe their privacy has been violated.
- Include contact information for an individual to obtain further information or make complaints.

If an individual's PHI is inaccurate or incomplete, under the HIPAA Privacy Rule, an individual has the right to request that the covered entity amend or correct the information. It also gives individuals the right to know when—and to whom—their PHI has been disclosed by a covered entity or a business associate. Under the HIPAA Privacy Rule, individuals also have the right to request restrictions on disclosure to persons involved in their health care or payment for their health care, or to notify family members or others about the individual's general condition, location, or death. However, a covered entity is under no obligation to agree to these requests. Finally, under the HIPAA Privacy Rule, health plans and covered health care providers must permit individuals to request an alternative means or location for receiving communications of protected health information.

The individual rights conveyed by the HIPAA Privacy Rule are a very significant part of the protections offered by HIPAA. While this section introduced these rights, Chapter 2 will present a more in-depth review of the individual rights established by the HIPAA Privacy Rule. It will also offer concrete advice on how to exercise those rights.

Permissible Uses and Disclosures of Health Information

HIPAA allows covered entities to use and disclose PHI for a variety of purposes without the prior consent of—or even prior notice to—an individual.[10] It should be emphasized that the categories of permitted uses and disclosures outlined below are indeed just that, permitted. In other words, they identify circumstances under which a covered entity would be *allowed* to use and/or disclose your PHI without your consent or knowledge. A covered entity is not *required* to use or disclose your PHI for these purposes.

Treatment, payment, and health care operations: This category enables a covered entity to use and/or disclose your PHI in a wide variety of ways, all in connection with your treatment, the payment for your care, and for their health care operations. This is a very wide category that can include different type of uses and disclosures. For example, this category would permit a covered entity to disclose PHI to a company that manages its databases as part of the covered entity's health care operations (provided, of course, that a business associate agreement is in place). It would also enable a covered entity to use and disclose PHI in order to receive payment for medical services rendered by the entity.

Required by law: A covered entity may disclose PHI when another law requires the disclosure of the information. So, be aware that if another law requires that your PHI be disclosed, a covered entity may not be able to protect the privacy of that PHI by asserting that HIPAA protects the requested PHI. For example, if a covered entity is under investigation for its billing practices and is required to disclose patient records in connection with the investigation, this category would permit the covered entity to do so.

Public health activities: Many different organizations and covered entities have an important role to play in assisting authorities with monitoring and protecting public health. As such, covered entities are sometimes called upon to disclose information relevant to public health to federal, state, and local public health agencies. As a good example of how this category may come into play, consider when in 2009, physicians were recently required to report H1N1 cases to governmental agencies.

While public health disclosures may often entail reporting information to governmental agencies, disclosures related to public health can also involve disclosures to private entities. For example, a physician may report adverse reactions to particular medications to the applicable pharmaceutical company. In some instances, disclosures to patients' employers may also qualify as permitted public health disclosures.

Victims of abuse, neglect, or domestic violence: Covered entities are able to use PHI to report on victims to police, social service organizations, and others who are authorized to receive such reports. For example, the HIPAA Privacy Rule would not restrict a covered entity from contacting police and reporting on the injuries of a domestic abuse victim who sought care in the emergency room.

Health oversight activities: Covered entities may also use and disclose PHI for health oversight activities that are authorized by law, such as audits, investigations, inspections, and so forth. Various state and federal agencies may oversee the functions of covered entities. This provision allows covered entities to disclose PHI to these agencies in connection with the oversight activities.

Judicial and administrative proceedings: Covered entities may also use PHI in connection with judicial and administrative proceedings, such as to respond to a court order, the order of an administrative agency, or subpoenas and discovery requests. The HIPAA Privacy Rule does, however, impose complicated conditions upon entities seeking to disclose PHI for such purposes. Their complexity is increased by the fact that they also interplay with other state and federal laws, as well as the rules of court. Attorneys sorting through these various conditions, rules, and requirements have quite a difficult task. For our purposes as consumers, it is important to make note of the fact that, despite the privacy protections afforded by the HIPAA Privacy Rule, your PHI may be shared if the covered entity needs to disclose it to respond to a judicial and/or administrative proceeding.

Law enforcement purposes: The HIPAA Privacy Rule allows covered entities to use and disclose PHI for a wide range of law enforcement purposes. For example, the police may be able to obtain information about a suspect's injuries in connection with the investigation of a crime.

Decedents: Covered entities can share PHI concerning a person who has died with coroners and funeral directors. These parties may need certain PHI, such as information about the deceased's cause of death and any diseases from which the decedent may have suffered.

Organ and tissue donation: The HIPAA Privacy Rule allows covered entities to disclose PHI to organizations involved with tissue banking and transportation.

Research: Covered entities are allowed to disclose PHI to those engaged in health research, but the research in question is generally required to have been approved by an institutional review board.

Serious threats to health or safety: A covered entity may disclose PHI if it has a good-faith belief that it is necessary to prevent or lessen a serious and imminent threat to the health or safety of a person or the public. For example, a physician might contact law enforcement authorities if she believed that one of her patients has a medical disorder that may make the person homicidal, or that same physician might contact a patient's wife if the patient had a medical condition that made it unsafe for him to drive but that patient continued to drive, thus jeopardizing the welfare of their children and others on the roads.

Specialized government functions: This category permits covered entities to use and disclose PHI for a variety of specialized government functions, including certain activities related to military, veterans, prison functions, and public benefit programs provided by the government.

National security or intelligence agency: This broad category allows a covered entity to respond to a request from any national security or intelligence agency for PHI without violating the HIPAA Privacy Rule.

Workers' compensation: The HIPAA Privacy Rule permits the use and disclosure of PHI where necessary to comply with laws concerning workers' compensation.

Administrative Requirements

The requirements of HIPAA reflect a recognition that covered entities range from small providers to the large multistate health plans. The HIPAA Privacy Rule allows covered entities to analyze their own needs and implement solutions appropriate for their own environment. What is appropriate for a particular covered entity will depend on the nature of its business, as well as its size and resources. There is a lot of flexibility built into HIPAA, particularly with respect to the HIPAA Security Rule that will be discussed in more detail in Chapter 3. Following are the key administrative requirements under the HIPAA Privacy Rule.

Privacy policies and procedures: A covered entity must develop and implement written privacy policies and procedures that are consistent with the HIPAA Privacy Rule.[11]

Privacy personnel: A covered entity must designate a privacy official responsible for developing and implementing privacy policies and procedures. It must also designate a contact person or contact office responsible for receiving complaints and providing individuals with information on the covered entity's privacy practices.

Workforce training and management: All workforce members must be trained by a covered entity on privacy policies and procedures as necessary and appropriate for them to carry out their duties. A covered entity must also have and apply appropriate sanctions against workforce members who violate the HIPAA Privacy Rule or its own privacy policies. Workforce members include employees, volunteers, trainees, and may also include others whose conduct is under the direct control of the entity (whether or not they are paid by the entity).[12]

Mitigation: A covered entity must mitigate, to the extent practicable, any harmful effect it learns was caused by use or disclosure of PHI by its workforce or its business associates in violation of its privacy policies and procedures or the HIPAA Privacy Rule.

Data safeguards: Reasonable and appropriate administrative, technical, and physical safeguards must be maintained by a covered entity in order to prevent use or disclosure of PHI in violation of the HIPAA Privacy Rule. Such safeguards might include shredding documents containing PHI before discarding them, securing medical records with lock and key or pass code, and limiting access to keys or pass codes.

Complaints: A covered entity must have procedures for individuals to complain about its compliance with its privacy policies and procedures and the HIPAA Privacy Rule. The covered entity must explain those procedures in its privacy practices notice. Among other things, the notice must identify to whom individuals can submit complaints to the covered entity and advise that complaints also can be submitted to the HHS secretary.

Retaliation and waiver: If a person exercises his or her rights under the HIPAA Privacy Rule, assists in an investigation, or voices opposition to an act or practice he or she believes violates the Privacy Rule, a covered entity is forbidden from retaliating. In addition, a covered entity may not require an individual to waive any right under the Privacy Rule as a condition for obtaining treatment, payment, and enrollment or benefits eligibility.

Documentation and record retention: The HIPAA Privacy Rule also imposes recordkeeping requirements. Specifically, a covered entity must maintain its privacy policies and procedures, its privacy practices notices, disposition of complaints and other actions, activities, and designations that the Privacy Rule requires to be documented for six years.

Fully insured group health plan exception: A fully insured group health plan that has no more than enrollment data and summary health information is only required to comply with the (1) ban on retaliatory acts and waiver of individual rights, and (2) documentation requirements of plan documents when the documents permit disclosure of PHI to the plan sponsor by a health insurance issuer or an HMO that services the group health plan.

The HIPAA Security Rule

The HIPAA Security Rule,[13] which became effective two years after the HIPAA Privacy Rule, is designed to protect the security of electronic health information. This is a very important point to emphasize. While the HIPAA Privacy Rule applies to PHI in any form, including oral communication, the HIPAA Security Rule applies only to PHI that is in electronic form, requiring that entities implement administrative, physical, and technical safeguards to protect PHI. Administrative standards include risk analysis and management; assigning security responsibilities, policies, and procedures; training of the workforce; and contract requirements. Physical safeguards include access to facilities and workstations, as well as device and media controls. Technical safeguards include access controls and audits, authentication, and transmission security.

The HIPAA Security Rule imposes standards that describe what must be done and implementation specifications that describe how the standards can be met. Implementation specifications are further divided into two groups: those that are required (e.g., risk analysis) and those that are "addressable" (e.g., encryption for transmission of PHI). If an entity chooses not to implement an addressable specification, it must document the reasons why, and, if reasonable and appropriate, implement alternative measures. In addition, like the Privacy Rule, the HIPAA Security Rule sets only the minimum data security standards that covered entities and their business associates must meet; those entities often face more stringent obligations under state law. States like Massachusetts and Nevada have enacted stringent data security laws that, while not geared specifically toward health information, would still cover some information that a covered entity and/or its business associate may possess, such as an individual's name and Social Security number.

While the HIPAA Security Rule is quite detailed and comprehensive, it does have a number of limitations. As with the HIPAA Privacy Rule, only certain organizations are required to comply with the HIPAA Security Rule. The original Security Rule applied only to covered entities. While the recently enacted HITECH Act (which will be discussed further below) requires business associates to also comply with most of the Security Rule, there are others—like personal health record vendors (discussed in Chapter 4)—that may have access to private information but fall outside the reach of the Security Rule.

In addition, as noted above, the HIPAA Security Rule protects only electronic medical records; it does not require covered entities to implement any security protections for health information stored in paper records. While there is an ongoing effort to implement electronic health records, many health records now exist only in paper form. The detailed requirements of the HIPAA Security Rule do not apply to these paper records, thus raising the question as to whether these records will be adequately protected.

Perhaps most importantly, the HIPAA Security Rule has not yet been vigorously enforced, according to research and government studies. The Centers for Medicare & Medicaid Services (CMS), which administers Medicare, Medicaid, and the Children's Health Insurance Program, received 378 security complaints as of 2008 without issuing any fines or penalties. "CMS [has] taken limited steps to ensure that covered entities adequately implement security protection," an October 2008 report by the HHS Inspector General said. "CMS ha[s] no effective mechanism to ensure that covered entities [are] complying with the HIPAA Security Rule or that ePHI [is] being adequately protected."[14]

This may be changing. In 2008, HHS entered into a resolution agreement with Seattle-based Providence Health & Services to resolve allegations of violations of the HIPAA Privacy and Security Rules in connection with the company's widely publicized losses of laptops and other sensitive items in 2005 and 2006. The settlement required Providence Health & Services to pay $100,000 and to implement a corrective action plan to ensure electronic patient information is appropriately safeguarded against future security breaches.[15] In addition, earlier in 2008, CMS partnered with PricewaterhouseCoopers to conduct security audits of some covered entities to examine if they were meeting the HIPAA Security Rule standards.[16] Finally, with new data breach notification obligations being mandated by the HITECH Act, regulators will have more information about breaches when they occur, and may very well take more legal actions against companies that fail to secure medical information.

The HITECH Act

In response to concerns over the recession, on February 17, 2009, President Obama signed into law the American Recovery and Reinvestment Act of 2009 (ARRA), known to many as the federal stimulus package.[17] While the stimulus package received much attention for its tax and spending provisions, the legislation also made significant changes to aspects of health care regulation, particularly the privacy and security of health information. Title XIII of ARRA, the Health Information Technology for Economic and Clinical Health Act (HITECH Act),[18] dedicated $22 billion in federal funding to advance the use of health information technology. Recognizing that effective data privacy and security is a necessary prerequisite to the digitization of our health care system, Subtitle D of the HITECH Act also modified many of HIPAA's privacy and security provisions in ways that are discussed further in the following sections.

Business Associates Are Subject to HIPAA

The HITECH Act makes business associates directly subject to many of HIPAA's requirements, as well as to the penalties for violating those requirements (before the act, only covered entities to which business associates provide services were subject to the rules). This expansion of the government's jurisdiction on HIPAA enforcement is a dramatic shift from former policy. Prior to the HITECH Act, business associates were not directly governed by HIPAA. Instead, they were governed only by the contracts (that HIPAA mandated they sign) with the covered entities they were doing business with. As such, a business associate who failed to comply with HIPAA's security or privacy requirements would face only the threat of contractual liability, not direct enforcement action by regulators. Under the changes ushered in by the HITECH Act, business associates will now be subject to the same government civil and criminal penalties as covered entities.

In addition to this significant shift, the HITECH Act also subjects business associates to a number of the substantive provisions of the regulations, including the requirements to implement administrative, physical, and technical safeguards to protect PHI. Business associates must also now comply with the HIPAA regulations requiring the implementation of formal policies and procedures as well as documentation requirements.

Although the HITECH Act directly regulates the conduct of business associates, they are still required to enter into contractual agreements with covered entities to which they provide services. These contracts, whether new or already in existence, must reflect the policy shift described above. In addition, any organization that transmits PHI to a covered entity or its business associate and requires routine access to such PHI will be required to enter into the appropriate business associate agreement with the covered entity and will be considered a business associate. The same holds true for vendors that contract with a covered entity to offer personal health records to individuals as part of the covered entity's electronic health records offering.

New Data Breach-Notification Requirements

Prior to the HITECH Act, while the majority of states had breach notification laws for data that can be used to commit financial identity theft, few extended the same requirements to health information. Moreover, until the HITECH Act, there was not any national law imposing data breach notification obligations. But the HITECH Act changed that by introducing the first federal breach-notification requirement.

The notification requirements under the HITECH Act apply to HIPAA covered entities and business associates, as well as vendors of personal health records. While following the lead of state-level data breach notification laws, the breach-notification requirements of the HITECH Act are much broader, as they cover any kind of personal information held by health care companies—names, addresses, contact information, and any other individually identifiable information, whether directly about the individual's "health" or not. By contrast, most state laws apply only to specific categories of information—such as Social Security numbers—where a breach could lead to identity theft.

Under the HITECH Act, covered entities will be required to notify individuals upon any compromise of their unsecured PHI, and business associates will be required to notify covered entities of such a breach. The breach notification must be made without unreasonable delay and within no more than 60 days following the detection of the breach. Furthermore, if the breach involves the data of more than 500 individuals, the covered entity must notify HHS as well as "prominent media outlets" in the applicable area. HHS will then post the details of these large breaches on its Web site for public viewing, and any covered entity that suffers a large breach of this nature will be required to maintain a log of such breaches to be submitted annually to HHS.

However, the breach-notification requirements of the HITECH Act do include critical, if limited, exceptions. First, the requirements apply only to "unsecured" information, defined as PHI that is "not secured through the use of a technology or methodology specified by the Secretary" and "not secured by a technology standard that renders protected health information unusable, unreadable, or indecipherable to unauthorized individuals" that has been developed or endorsed by an accredited organization.[19] Per HHS, "secured" information includes "encrypted" information meeting certain technical standards, as well as "destroyed" information. This exception should motivate entities to pursue expanded uses of encryption as the means for protecting the PHI that they possess.

In addition, the statute creates an exception where the unauthorized recipient "would not reasonably have been able to retain the information."[20] Such a case might include when a health care provider mails information to the wrong individual and it is returned to the post office because of the incorrect address.[21] In such an instance, the recipient, although not authorized to view the information, was not able to retain it and, therefore, it is not a breach.

While the HITECH Act established the general rules applicable to data breach responses, it also required HHS and the Federal Trade Commission (FTC) to adopt rules to govern the particular entities under their jurisdiction. For the FTC, this means PHR vendors and related entities, and for the HHS, this means covered entities and their business associates.

The FTC Rule

The HITECH Act required the FTC to create a breach-notification rule covering personal health record vendors, many of whom are not otherwise covered by HIPAA. Personal health records will be discussed in detail in Chapter 4. For now, however, it is worthwhile to review the key provisions of the breach-notification rules applicable to the entities that are involved with the provisions of these types of health records. The FTC issued its regulation (the FTC Rule) on August 17, 2009,[22] and it focuses on two kinds of entities: (1) vendors of personal health records[23] (companies that provide repositories that people can use to keep track of their health information) and (2) entities that offer third-party applications for personal health records (including devices, like pedometers or blood pressure monitors, that produce readings consumers can upload into their personal health records).

The FTC Rule applies to a limited class of entities, namely personal health record vendors that are not subject to HIPAA and their service providers. In fact, the rule makes clear that (with very limited exceptions) the FTC's jurisdiction extends only to entities that are outside HHS jurisdiction under HIPAA. This way, companies face only one regulator for these issues, and consumers receive only one notice in the event of a security breach.

While advocates of greater health privacy regulation may be disappointed that public health record vendors are not subject to more stringent privacy and/or data security requirements in the new legislation, this breach-notification rule represents the first step in the regulation of these entities and mandates a future study to consider a broader set of restrictions on the activities of these entities.

The FTC rule does not preempt state breach-notification laws. Accordingly, entities covered by the FTC rule must comply with both that rule and any relevant state laws. Given the Web-based business model of most personal health record vendors, this dual compliance obligation seems likely to remain a substantial source of complications when breaches occur. This could be bad for consumers as well, as there are justifiable concerns over the concept of over-notification and the impact this could have on consumers' perceptions of the gravity of breaches involving their PHI, as well as their responses to breach notices.

The FTC rule creates a rebuttable presumption that unauthorized *access* to personal health record information leads to the unauthorized *acquisition* of that information, but provides the opportunity for regulated entities to demonstrate that the unauthorized access *did not* lead to improper acquisition. This kind of situation may occur for example, if a laptop is stolen but a forensic analysis indicates that the laptop password was not breached and no information was viewed.

However, the FTC did not accept the proposal that it should require notification only in the even that there is a risk of harm. This, as we shall see in the next section, is an important distinction between the FTC rule and the rule passed by HHS.

The FTC rule is effective for breaches that take place 30 days after publication in the *Federal Register*.[24] That publication occurred on August 25, 2009, and the rule's stated effective date is September 24, 2009. However, the FTC was sympathetic to industry concerns about the effects of this rule and has indicated that it would not to seek penalties for compliance failures until February 22, 2010. At the time of this writing, the FTC had not commenced any enforcement actions for violations of the FTC rule. However, given the FTC's high level of activity in enforcing data security obligations in other areas[25] one might speculate that actions may very well be forthcoming.

The HHS Rule

Under the HITECH Act, like the FTC, HHS was also required to develop a specific rule for how covered entities and their business associates must handle notifications of breaches involving PHI. The HHS regulation was developed by that agency's Office of Civil Rights, the enforcement agency for the HIPAA Privacy Rule, and—in a recent development—the HIPAA Security Rule. It was released on August 19, 2009, as an "Interim Final Rule," and was published in the August 24, 2009, *Federal Register* (the "HHS Rule").[26] The stated effective date was September 23, 2009. Just prior to the publication of this book, HHS quietly withdrew the HHS Rule for further consideration. There has been some speculation that the further consideration of the HHS Rule might result in a rule that is even more protective of privacy rights. In particular, there has been some suggestion that HHS might revisit the "risk of harm" test that was included in the HHS Rule but not the FTC Rule.

While the FTC rule applies to a relatively limited set of entities, the HHS rule applies across the health care industry to all covered entities and their business associates. The bulk of the rule deals with the details of notice about breaches—the notice's timing, its content, and how the entities will communicate to HHS and the media about breaches. Beyond these largely procedural requirements, there are a number of points about the HHS rule that merit deeper analysis.

First, under the HITECH Act, notification is required only for breaches involving "unsecured" information. In its proposed rule, HHS identified encryption and "destruction" of information as appropriate means of securing information that would not require reporting. In the final regulation, HHS reviewed and then rejected various additional means of securing information. Accordingly, to take advantage of this "safe harbor," companies must encrypt or destroy information. HHS was quite explicit as to the distinction between appropriate and effective security practices and this safe harbor. For example, HHS directly addressed the concern of some in the health care industry over potentially mandatory encryption by clarifying that there is no encryption mandate, that it is just the approach that allows a company to take advantage of this notification safe harbor. While other security measures (redaction, limited data sets, etc.) may be effective to reduce any risk of a breach in the first place or the potential harm from a breach, they will not, by themselves, eliminate the duty to notify of a breach.

One of the biggest concerns that many covered entities expressed over the breach notification provisions of the HITECH Act was that companies would be required to provide notice of all breaches, including those in which there was no risk of any harm to the consumer whose information was breached. Covered entities noted the costs and other concerns stemming from such disclosures, while consumer advocates worried that these notices could cause undue concern, confusion, or fear. Unlike the FTC, HHS implemented a realistic and responsible "risk of harm" threshold, requiring notice when the breach "poses a significant risk of financial, reputational, or other harm to the individual." The burden of determining that there is no "significant risk" falls on the covered entity, which otherwise is responsible for notifying the affected individual. Due to the considerable criticism that HHS has faced over the inclusion of the "risk of harm" test, it is possible that this might be one of the aspects of the HHS Rule that is changed as a result of HHS' further consideration of the HHS Rule.

The HHS rule also includes some interesting discussions about whether certain activities should be considered "breaches." On the one hand, HHS clarifies that only "impermissible" uses and disclosures under HIPAA qualify as breaches. This means, for example, that "incidental disclosures"—disclosures that may occur despite reasonable precautions, like one patient overhearing a doctor discuss an issue with another patient—are permitted under the HIPAA Privacy Rule and therefore do not qualify as breaches. On the other hand, HHS indicated that a disclosure of "more than" the minimum necessary information might be considered a breach. While covered entities still will apply the "risk of harm" threshold in this context, HHS has focused the industry's attention on some less obvious forms of potential breaches.

Like the FTC, HHS recognized many of the concerns about the reporting timetable. Accordingly, while HHS required compliance with this provision on the statutory timetable (30 days after publication of the rule in the *Federal Register*), it expressed that it would not issue penalties until February 22, 2010. The HHS was clear that this enforcement delay should not be construed as a delay in compliance. Accordingly, companies subject to the HHS rule have been required to comply with the rule since September 2009. HHS is expected to issue a new version of the HHS Rule. Until then, entities will need to comply with the version of the rule discussed herein.

Again, at the time of this writing, there had not been any federal enforcement actions arising out of a failure to notify consumers of a breach as required by the HITECH Act. However, as will be discussed further in Chapter 3, the Connecticut state Attorney General recently launched an enforcement action against a company that had experienced a breach of health-related data. This company's apparent delay in notifying consumers of the breach appeared to be a crucial factor for Connecticut's Attorney General. While this was the first action brought by a state attorney general under the new rules, it is unlikely that it will be the last. In fact, at the time of this writing, Connecticut's Attorney General was investigating a breach that occurred at Yale Medical School.

OTHER FEDERAL LAWS

Overview

Beyond HIPAA, there are several federal laws that impact the privacy and confidentiality of health information, including: (i) the Privacy Act of 1974;[27] (ii) the Confidentiality of Alcohol and Drug Abuse Patient Records Regulations;[28] (iii) the Family Educational Rights and Privacy Act (FERPA);[29] (iv) the Americans with Disabilities Act (ADA);[30] and (v) the Genetic Information Nondiscrimination Act of 2008 (GINA).[31] These key federal laws are highlighted below. Many of them will be discussed in further detail in subsequent chapters.

The Privacy Act of 1974

The Privacy Act of 1974 covers nearly all personal records (not just health records) maintained by federal agencies and some federal contractors. It applies to military health records, veterans' records, Indian Health Service records, Medicare records, and medical records of other federal agencies. (HIPAA also applies to these same federal records.) The Privacy Act of 1974 does not apply to most hospitals, clinics, or physicians, even if they receive federal funds or are tax-exempt. Generally speaking, the Privacy Act of 1974 grants people four rights: (i) to find out what information the government has collected about them; (ii) to see, and have, a copy of that information; (iii) to correct or amend that information; and (iv) to exercise limited control of the disclosure of that information to other parties.

Confidentiality of Alcohol and Drug Abuse Patient Records Regulations

The Confidentiality of Alcohol and Drug Abuse Patient Records Regulations (CADAPR Regulations), which were implemented in 1974, are another important set of federal laws. Specifically, the rules establish protections for the medical records of federally funded substance abuse programs. The Substance Abuse and Mental Health Services Administration (SAMHSA), a part of HHS, administers the alcohol and drug abuse rules. The CADAPR establish very strict rules regarding data privacy. In many respects, the rules are stricter than HIPAA, but when they are less stringent than HIPAA, the HIPAA Privacy Rule prevails. These CADAPR Regulations will be discussed further in Chapter 7. Generally, the regulations (i) describe the written summary and communication that must occur at the time of admission or as soon as the patient is capable of rational communication, relative to the confidentiality of alcohol and drug abuse patient records under federal law; (ii) define circumstances in which an individual's health information can be used and disclosed without patient authorization; (iii) require that each disclosure of health information be accompanied by specific language prohibiting redisclosure; (iv) do not prohibit patient access; (v) define the requirements of a written consent; and (vi) address who may consent on behalf of the patient.

The Family Educational Rights and Privacy Act

FERPA is a federal law codified in 1974 that protects the privacy of students' education records, which includes health records. The legislation applies to educational agencies and institutions that receive funds under any Department of Education program, including virtually all public schools and school districts and most private and public postsecondary institutions, including medical and other professional schools. If an educational agency or institution receives funds under one or more of these programs, FERPA applies to the entire parent organization, such as a department within a larger university or a single school in a district.

Subject to limited exceptions, FERPA prohibits covered educational agencies and institutions from disclosing student education records, or personally identifiable information from those records, without a parent or eligible student's written consent.

Records that are made, maintained, and used only in connection with the medical treatment of a student, and disclosed only to individuals providing the treatment, are excluded from the definition of "education records." These records are commonly called "treatment records." An eligible student's treatment records may be disclosed for purposes other than the student's treatment, provided the records are disclosed under one of the exceptions to written consent—or with the student's written consent. If a school discloses an eligible student's treatment records for purposes other than treatment, the records are no longer excluded from the definition of "education records" and are subject to all other FERPA requirements.

The Americans with Disabilities Act

The Americans with Disabilities Act of 1990 (ADA), which will be discussed further in Chapter 5 in relation to workplace privacy issues, is also worth mentioning here. The ADA prohibits job discrimination relating to physical or mental impairments that do not prevent an individual from performing work responsibilities when provided with "reasonable accommodation" by the employer.

Significantly, the ADA also establishes important confidentiality requirements for employee health information, requiring that medical information from physical examinations, questionnaires, or other means be obtained only *after* an offer of conditional employment. Such information must be obtained for all newly hired candidates, not just those with disabilities. Medical examinations of current employees are permitted to determine whether employees are "fit for duty" when safety is a concern and when required by federal, state, or local laws as long as the information obtained is not used in a way that violates the ADA. Examinations can also be performed as part of voluntary employee health programs subject to the same requirement of not violating the ADA.

The ADA requires that medical information be maintained in confidential files, separate from normal personnel files. Such information must not be disclosed to anyone other than managers and supervisors who need to know of work restrictions or accommodations, as well as: first aid and safety personnel to provide emergency services, government officials investigating compliance with the ADA, and workers' compensation offices in accordance with state laws.

While it seems that the ADA protects confidentiality in important ways, it has significant limitations. Since it does not restrict the types of health information that can be collected in employment-related physical examinations, a wide variety of PHI can be collected that is not directly job-related. It also does not provide guidelines to prevent managers from accessing and looking through all and any medical information in an employee's file while reviewing health information relevant to the employee's job-related fitness.

The Genetic Information Nondiscrimination Act

The Genetic Information Nondiscrimination Act of 2008 (GINA) provides federal protection from genetic discrimination in health insurance and employment. Genetic discrimination occurs when people are treated differently by their employer or insurance company because they have a genetic change that causes or increases the risk of an inherited disorder. Generally, GINA makes it illegal for health insurance providers to use or require genetic information to make decisions about a person's insurance eligibility or coverage and that person's hiring, promotion, and terms of employment. Given the connection between the restrictions of GINA and the workplace, GINA will be discussed further in Chapter 5 in connection with the discussion of health privacy at work.

With genetic testing capabilities improving and genetic testing becoming more widespread, the importance of this issue will likely only grow in the future. In fact, since 2002, the ability of genetic testing to determine predisposition to disease has increased by 12 percent annually.[32] In the future, a substantial part of the growth may be due to consumers who are seeking their own genetic tests. In many states, individuals have the ability to procure their own genetic testing as a way of managing their own health and predicting the health of any possible offspring.[33] To avoid any possible negative repercussions, including possible discrimination, individuals procuring these tests on their own will often want to secure the privacy of this data. At the same time, with continually rising health care costs and the need to maintain cost control, insurers, employers, and others may find this information of interest. This intrinsic tension will likely mean that the importance in protecting the privacy of genetic information will only continue to grow.

While GINA itself is rather comprehensive, many states have also enacted laws to prevent genetic discrimination. Accordingly, if genetic information privacy and nondiscrimination are of concern, like the other issues discussed in this book, it is essential to consult applicable state law in addition to federal law.

STATE LAWS

HIPAA's Privacy Rule establishes the minimum privacy protection for health information, while at the same time allowing more protective laws to exist at the state level. Covered entities are required to comply with both HIPAA and state law whenever possible, but some state provisions are preempted by HIPAA. However, state law is *not* preempted in the following circumstances: (i) when state law is necessary for regulation of insurance or health plans, prevention of fraud and abuse, or reporting on health care system operations and costs; (ii) when it addresses controlled substances; (iii) when it relates to reporting of disease or injury, child abuse, birth, or death, public health surveillance, or public health investigation or intervention; and (iv) when a provision of state law is more stringent than similar requirements in the HIPAA Privacy Rule.[34]

The most difficult of these exceptions to understand is the stringency exception. Generally, a provision of state law is considered more stringent if it prohibits or restricts use or disclosure of PHI that would be permitted under the HIPAA Privacy Rule. Specifically, a more stringent state law: (i) permits greater access and amendment rights to individuals; (ii) provides individuals with more information about use, disclosure, rights, and remedies; (iii) makes the requirement of legal permission for use or disclosure of PHI more lenient; (iv) increases the duration or requires more detailed accounting of disclosures; and (v) provides greater individual privacy protection.[35]

While these criteria should, in theory, provide guidance as to when state law is or isn't preempted by HIPAA, in practice it is not always clear. Although many health care companies and professional associations have undertaken their own analyses of the interaction between HIPAA and state law, these are only advisory in nature. There is general agreement that final decisions about the applicability of specific provisions of state and federal law is—and will continue to be—made by the courts.

State law is an increasingly important part of health privacy regulation. State laws cover health insurance regulation; the regulation of organizations that perform certain administrative functions, such as utilization review or third-party administration; licensure requirements for various medical specialties and medical organizations (including requirements for recordkeeping and disclosure); access to medical records; reporting of information to the state and local authorities; use of information for quality assurance and health care operations; issuance of notices of privacy practices; and reporting and providing access to law enforcement authorities.

As noted earlier in this book, in recent years many states have passed confidentiality laws related to specific conditions or types of health information. Examples include laws related to mental health records, HIV/AIDS, reproductive rights, and genetic testing. States may have laws concerning privacy in connection with insurance, workers compensation, public health, or research.

Meanwhile, states are also becoming increasingly involved with data security. Most states now have laws mandating the disclosure of breaches involving certain data and information that can be used to commit identity theft or other harm. While all of these state laws do extend to financial data, such as social security numbers and bank account numbers, a smaller number of states are beginning to extend their laws to cover breaches of medical and health information. In addition, certain states, including, most notably Massachusetts, have enacted comprehensive information security laws.

It is beyond the scope of this book to examine all such state laws in detail. However, ensuing chapters will discuss key relevant state laws. As a practical matter, given the fact that HIPAA largely sets the minimum for privacy protection and allows for more stringent laws at the state level, one should be aware of the need to always consult applicable state law when considering medical privacy.

CONCLUSION

This chapter has presented an introductory overview to significant privacy and data security laws in the health and medical sector. Clearly, it is a complicated playing field. While the primary instrument is HIPAA, as has been demonstrated, there are other federal laws and also state laws that play important roles in our health privacy. This legal framework will be explored further in the ensuing chapters as we examine the key issues under investigation.

Chapter 2 will drill down deeper into HIPAA, focusing on the individual rights conveyed by HIPAA. In addition to presenting and discussing these protections, this chapter will offer concrete advice on how individuals may exercise those rights. For example, in addition to explaining the meaning of the right to an accounting of disclosures of PHI, it will explain how to actually obtain an accounting of the disclosures of your medical information that have been made by your health care provider.

2

Your Rights under HIPAA and How to Exercise Them

INTRODUCTION

While the Health Insurance Portability and Accountability Act (HIPAA)[1] has been subject to a fair amount of criticism,[2] it is undeniable that the law does establish certain important individual rights. In practice, some of the rights will prove to be more valuable than others. However, in any event, all medical consumers should be well aware of the rights that they have under HIPAA and how they may exercise those rights. This chapter explores the individual rights that are established by HIPAA and offers advice on how those rights may be exercised.

YOUR RIGHTS UNDER HIPAA

Overview

Individuals have the following rights under the HIPAA Privacy Rule:[3] (i) the right of access to PHI; (ii) the right to amend PHI; (iii) the right to an accounting of disclosures; (iv) the right to receive privacy notices; (v) the right to request confidential communications; (vi) the right to request restrictions on uses or disclosures of PHI; and (vii) the right to file a complaint. The ensuing sections discuss each of these rights and the means for exercising them.

The Right of Access[4]

Overview of the Right of Access

With some exceptions, individuals have the right to access, inspect, and copy PHI held by covered entities. This is a very important right. There are many reasons why an individual may wish to exercise the right of access. For instance, you may feel that there are errors or inaccuracies in your file or you may suspect that you are a victim of identity theft. Also, having a copy of your medical records can be helpful if you wish to seek a second opinion from another doctor, especially if you do not want to have duplicate tests run and do not want your doctor to know that you are seeking a second opinion. Exercising the right to access health records can also be helpful if you wish to keep a copy of your health information in one place in your possession. Having access to your medical records can also be helpful if you believe that your insurance company improperly denied your claim. Also, if you feel a health care provider may have committed malpractice and you wish to discuss this with an attorney, obtaining your medical records in advance may help the attorney be in a better position to assess your case. These are just some examples of factors that may prompt a desire to access medical records. Of course, you may just be curious about what is in your medical record. Whatever the reason might be, the legislature recognized that this is a very strong interest that an individual would have, and therefore the rule affords the right to obtain one's medical records without a requirement to disclose any reason.

Limitations to the Right of Access

While the right of access is a broad right, it is not without its limits. As one notable exception to the right of access, patients do not have the right to access a provider's psychotherapy notes. Psychotherapy notes can generally be understood as notes taken by a mental health professional during a conversation with the patient and kept separate from the patient's medical and billing records.

In addition to the psychotherapy notes mentioned above, HIPAA's right of access also does not apply to materials compiled for litigation and records from non-CLIA[5] laboratories. A non-CLIA lab is generally one that performs research. For most patients, this will never be an issue. However, if your request for access for particular records is denied and the explanation is that the records come from a non-CLIA lab, this would be a permissible reason for the covered entity to withhold the records.

A covered entity can also deny your request to access certain records, including records maintained by a prison, some records of research participants, and records obtained from someone other than a health care provider under a promise of confidentiality. Furthermore, a covered entity can deny you access to certain records if a licensed health professional determines that such access is reasonably likely to endanger the life or physical safety of you or another individual. A covered entity can also refuse to provide access to a patient's representative if disclosure would cause substantial harm.

If a covered entity withholds records for any of these reasons, it must provide a written denial explaining the reason for the denial. It must also explain any appeal rights that you have.

Exercising the Right of Access

If you wish to request access to records, you should start by reviewing the applicable covered entity's notice of privacy practices. If correctly drafted, this notice will describe your right to access and obtain a copy of your medical record. It should also describe the procedures for exercising this right. In most cases, you will be asked to write a letter or fill in a form to exercise your right. A covered entity may insist upon a signed, written request. The covered entity may also ask you for identification to verify your identity. Sample Document 2.1 is a sample patient access request form. This form has been provided for illustrative purposes. You should always review the policies and procedures of the particular covered entity from which you are requesting your PHI.

The covered entity must respond to your request within 30 days.[6] This does not necessarily mean that you will have a copy of your records within 30 days. In fact, if the covered entity contacts you with a written explanation of the delay, the entity can take an additional 30 days to respond. If you need the records more quickly, you should convey this to the covered entity. The entity will not have an obligation to respond more quickly than what is required by law. However, depending on the situation, your covered entity may agree to respond more quickly.

The HITECH Act has introduced limited changes to the access right.[7] HIPAA does not specify the format in which the PHI must be provided. The HITECH Act has changed this for covered entities that utilize electronic health records. If a covered entity uses or maintains an electronic health record and an individual requests a copy of his or her PHI in electronic format, the covered entity must provide the requested PHI in electronic format to the person or entity that is clearly, conspicuously, and specifically designated by the individual.

Access Fees

Under HIPAA, individuals have both the right to access their health records and the right to copy their records. If you wish to secure a copy of your health records, the provider can charge a fee. However, if you simply wish to access and inspect the record, the covered entity cannot charge you to do so.

If you do seek to obtain copies of your medical records, the covered entity can charge a reasonable, cost-based fee for copying and postage. With respect to electronic copies of PHI, the HITECH Act specifies that a covered entity must limit its charges to the labor costs incurred in responding to the request. Furthermore, state law may establish lower fees than HIPAA permits. When asked to pay fees for your medical records, review the proposed charge carefully to ensure that you are not being charged more than what is permissible under HIPAA or applicable state law.

While, as noted, HIPAA permits covered entities to charge only a reasonable fee, these costs can add up quite quickly. Copying costs can be $1 per page or more. In addition, if seeking copies of other records, such as x-rays, the fees can be even higher. If you consider the size of a typical medical file, you can imagine how the copying costs can add up, especially if you are seeking to copy all files for a number of doctors over a multi-year period. If you are switching doctors and have a serious medical issue, for example, you may feel you need a copy of your entire medical file. On the other hand, you may be able to limit your search to records concerning a particular procedure or a particular set of records, for instance, those concerning your prescriptions. Accordingly, unless you require your entire medical file, it will be in your best interest to narrow your search. This will help to cut costs dramatically. In addition, copies of electronic records can be less expensive to acquire. Accordingly, if your covered entity already maintains electronic records, it may be far more cost-effective to obtain electronic records. In addition, as noted above, if you wish to verify information but do not actually need copies, you can request the right to access and review your records without obtaining a copy.

If you do not believe that the fees that are being charged are permissible, try to resolve your concerns with the applicable covered entity. If that fails, you can file a complaint with the Department of Health and Human Services (HHS). The process for filing complaints is discussed further in this chapter. In addition, if you require a copy of the records but cannot afford to pay, you may wish to ask for a waiver. Some covered entities may provide waivers or fee reductions.

A Word about State Law

This summary has focused upon the rights of access that are established by HIPAA. As noted, HIPAA only establishes the floor of protection. Accordingly, it is possible that your state's law may grant you greater access rights. For example, HIPAA provides covered entities with a longer period to respond to a patient's access request than some state laws. New York law requires that if a provider has space to permit visual inspection of medical records, it must permit visual inspection of records within 10 days and furnish a copy within a reasonable time. Otherwise, if the provider does not have space to allow on-site visual inspection, the provider must provide a copy within 10 days.[8] Similarly, in California, an individual is allowed to inspect his or her medical records during the health care provider's business hours within five working days after the provider receives the individual's written access request. Accordingly, when attempting to exercise your right to access your medical records, you should first review the provider's notice of privacy practices in order to understand the provider's explanation of the processes for obtaining access to medical records, but you should also investigate applicable state law to see whether it grants you any greater rights than you are afforded under HIPAA.

The Right to Amend[9]

Overview

Individuals have the right to request amendments to PHI held by covered entities. Upon accessing and reviewing your medical records, you may discover that those records contain information that does not belong to you, are missing information that is important to your care, or contain inaccurate information. In such a case, you would have a right to request an amendment of your health record.

Exercising Your Right to Amend

Before attempting to exercise your right to pursue an amendment to your medical records, you should do your own research and get prepared. Specifically, before asking for an amendment to your medical records, you should obtain copies of the records, review them, and identify the part(s) that is believed to be inaccurate or incomplete. You should then identify the provider who created that information and/or was responsible for placing that information in your medical record in the first place. Then, you should contact that provider to determine if they have a specific procedure for requesting amendments. Many health care providers will have their own form for requesting amendments. If they do have their own form, you are advised to use it, as it may streamline the process. Under the HIPAA Privacy Rule, a provider may require that you submit your amendment request in writing, but must advise you in advance that it is a requirement. The health care provider can also require that you provide a reason for why you are seeking an amendment.

Some health care providers may not supply their own forms for requesting medical records. In this case, you may save time, and the possible need to redo your efforts, by contacting the provider in advance to see what they require. The provider's notice of privacy practices may contain the details about how you may exercise your amendment right. Generally, an amendment request should include: (i) your name; (ii) your address; (iii) your telephone number; (iv) your e-mail address; (v) your medical record identification number (if you know it) and/or other identifiers, such as date of birth or social security number;[10] (vi) date(s) of service; (vii) the type of information that you wish to amend; (viii) a description of the information that you believe is inaccurate or incomplete; (ix) the information that you wish to add to your record, if any; and (x) the reason why you wish to add the information.

It is important to note that the HIPAA Privacy Rule does not allow you to have information removed from your record, it only provides the right to

SAMPLE DOCUMENT 2.1: PATIENT REQUEST FOR ACCESS TO MEDICAL RECORDS

Authorization for Release of Protected Health Information (PHI)
(*Required Information)

*Name of Patient: _____

*Soc. Security #: _____

*Address: _____

*Phone Number: _____

*Date of Birth: _____

E-mail Address: _____

Medical Record #: _____

1. **Type of Request:** I hereby request that _____ (hospital or physician) provide the health records described in this authorization.

2. **Reason for Release:** ☐ Personal Copy ☐ Transfer to New Doctor ☐ Move ☐ Attorney/Legal ☐ Insurance

3. ***Select delivery method:** ☐ Pick up in Person ☐ U.S. Mail ☐ Certified Overnight Delivery (Extra Charge) ☐ eRelease ☐ Other (method) _____

4. **Date Range of Health Records to be Released:** _____

5. ***Description of Records to be Released:**
   _____
   _____

6. **Specific Confidential PHI Authorized for This Release:**
   I am authorizing _____(hospital or physician) to release the indicated type of information pursuant to this authorization from the treatment date(s) listed above.
   _____
   _____

7. ***Release of PHI.** I request that you release my PHI to:
   _____ Patient (Same as Above)
   _____Parent/guardian/organization/insurance/lawyer, etc.
   Name: _____
   Address: _____
   E-mail: _____

8. **Fees**: I understand I may incur a reasonable, cost-based fee where applicable for copying from microfilm, postage, preparation, and labor.
   _____ I agree to pay all charges.
   _____ Please contact me with the estimated full cost before proceeding.

9. **Expiration Date.** This signed authorization will expire in one year unless an earlier date is indicated. Alternate date (if applicable):_____

10. Revocation of Authorization: I understand that I may revoke this authorization by sending a letter to _____ (name of health care provider) at the address listed above.

By my signature below, I acknowledge and agree that I have read and agree to the terms of this authorization.

_____
Signature

_____
Name

_____
Date

_____
Relationship to patient

add more information. Furthermore, it does not provide any right to require your provider to change a diagnosis with which you may disagree. However, if your provider has made a diagnosis with which you disagree and you have additional information to add to your records, which you do through exercising your right to amend, this may impact how the diagnosis that is contained in your records may be interpreted.

The covered entity must respond to your request for an amendment. As we will see below, this is not to say that they have to honor the request—but they must respond to it. Generally, the covered entity must respond within 60 days after the receipt of the request. However, if the applicable covered entity is unable to act within the mandated 60-day period, it can get a single 30-day extension. In order to get this extension, however, the covered entity must give you a written explanation for the delay and also advise as to the date upon which they expect to respond, which should not be longer than a total of 90 days.

If the covered entity accepts your request to amend your medical record, they must add the new information to your record. If you know of third parties who should be made aware of the amendments to your medical records, you should provide the names and contact information for those individuals, companies, and/or organizations to the applicable covered entity that has made the amendment. The applicable covered entity must then give the amended health information to the people and organizations you identify. Sample Document 2.2 illustrates an example of a sample amendment request.

A covered entity may deny an amendment request. Generally, the request can be denied when (i) the covered entity determines that your record is accurate or complete, or (ii) the covered entity did not create the information that you wish to amend. If the covered entity denies your amendment request, they must inform you in writing and must also explain why your request was denied. Sample Document 2.3 illustrates an example of how a denial notice may appear. If the covered entity does not agree to your request, you have the right to submit a statement of disagreement that the health care provider or plan must add to your record. The covered entity may disagree with your statement, but they must still include the statement in your file. They can, however, also include in your file a note explaining why they disagree with you. The covered entity must provide you with a copy of this note.

As noted, your amendment right extends to the covered entity that has created the medical record at issue. This begs the question of what is to be done in situations in which the applicable covered entity is no longer around. This is a very real possibility when one is dealing with a covered entity that is a sole practitioner. If you do find yourself in this situation, you should explain to the current holder of your medical records, with as much detail as possible, that the provider who created the original record is no longer available to act on your request.

The Impact of State Law

Some states add to the federal amendment right that was established by HIPAA. For example, California law permits individuals to write a short statement explaining their side of the story, so to speak, and submit to their provider so that this statement can be added to one's medical record, even where the amendment request is permitted.[11] While writing such a statement may seem like a simpler approach, some may feel that pursuing an amendment of PHI under the rights established by HIPAA and having the covered entity make the change may give the change more credibility.

The Right to Accounting[12]

Overview

HIPAA established that individuals have the right to request accountings of disclosures of their PHI that have been made by the covered entity. With respect to disclosures of PHI, an "accounting" is a record (i) of the date the PHI was disclosed; (ii) the name of the person or entity receiving the PHI; (iii) a brief description of the PHI disclosed; and (iv) a brief statement of the purpose of the disclosure.

Many individuals may never need or want to make a request for an accounting of the disclosure of their PHI. However, there are certain circumstances under which this right can become important. For example, if you feel you have been the victim of medical identity theft, you may make a request for an accounting to see if you might be able to track down for yourself where the information may have been compromised. Of course, you may also wish to make a request out of pure curiosity and a wish to better understand to whom your medical records are circulated.

SAMPLE DOCUMENT 2.2: PATIENT REQUEST FOR AMENDMENT/ CORRECTION OF PHI

Patient Name: _____ Request Date: _____

Street Address: _____ Birth Date: _____

City/State/Zip: _____ Account #: _____

What Needs to be Amended/Corrected and Why

Entry to be amended: _____

Date and author of entry: _____

Please explain how the information is incorrect or incomplete. What should the information state to be more accurate or complete?

_____

_____

_____

_____

Would you like this amendment sent to anyone to whom we may have disclosed this information in the past? If so, please specify the name and address of the organization or individual.

_____

_____

Names and addresses:

_____

_____

I understand that the provider may or may not amend the medical record with an amendment based on my request, and under no circumstances is the provider permitted to alter the original medical record. In any event, this request for an amendment will be made part of my permanent medical record.

Signature of Patient or Patient's Legal Representative: _____

Date: _____

For Health Care Organization/Internal Use Only

Date received: _____

Accepted _____ Denied _____

If denied, check reason for denial:

☐ PHI was not created by this organization

☐ PHI is not available to the patient for inspection as permitted by federal law (e.g., psychotherapy notes)

☐ PHI is not part of patient's designated record set

☐ PHI is accurate and complete

Comments:

Individual was informed of denial in writing (attach letter of communication)

_____   _____

Signature/title of staff member   Date

**SAMPLE DOCUMENT 2.3: SAMPLE LETTER DENYING
A REQUEST FOR AMENDMENT**

Name:
Address 1:
Address 2:

Date:
Re: Request for Amendment to Medical Record # _____

Dear Patient:
Thank you for submitting to us your request for amendment/correction of health information. Your request was forwarded to the _____ (designated official) for review.

Your request has been denied for the following reason(s):

☐ The information was not created by this organization.
☐ The information is not available to you for inspection as permitted by federal law (e.g., psychotherapy notes).
☐ The information is not part of your designated record set.
☐ The information is accurate and complete.

If you disagree with this denial, you may file a written statement of disagreement with the (define appropriate organizational contact/office here). Please limit your statement to one typewritten page or two handwritten pages. If you choose not to file a statement of disagreement, you may request that we include your request for amendment/correction of health information, as well as this denial of your request, with any future disclosures of the protected health information that is the subject of the requested amendment.

If you feel that you would like to file a complaint with the Secretary of the federal Department of Health and Human Services, you can address your complaint to 200 Independence Avenue, S.W., Washington, DC 20201, or reach the Secretary by phone at (202) 690-7000.

Sincerely,
HIPAA Privacy Officer

Under HIPAA, the right to an accounting is extended to all disclosures made without authorization to anyone other than the individual for purposes other than treatment, payment, and health care operations in the six years prior to the individual's request for an accounting. However, the HITECH Act has expanded the accounting right. The expansion is related to the increasing use of electronic health records (EHRs). Under HIPAA, covered entities were not required to account for disclosures made for treatment, payment, and health care operations. The theory was that covered entities need to make a number of routine disclosures for treatment, payment, and health care operations, and requiring the entity to account for all of these routine disclosures would be unduly burdensome and time-consuming for the covered entity. Technology will make the tracking and accounting of such disclosures less burdensome, however. Accordingly, under the HITECH Act, if a covered entity utilizes an EHR, such covered entity will be required to account for such disclosures for treatment, payment, and health care operations. For such requests, the covered entity will need to account for disclosures occurring within the three years prior to the date of the request.

This new requirement is being implemented in a staggered manner. For covered entities that had an EHR as of January 1, 2009, the effective date for implementing the new accounting rule is January 1, 2014, and for covered entities that acquire an EHR after January 1, 2009, the effective date is the later of January 1, 2011, or the date the EHR is acquired. The HHS Secretary is empowered to delay these effective dates by two years if necessary.

The deadline disparity, while seemingly counterintuitive, is based upon the assumption that EHRs acquired before January 1, 2009, are not likely to have the technical capacity to account for disclosures made for the purposes of treatment, payment, and health care operations. Accordingly, covered entities with EHRs in place prior to January 1, 2009, will have additional time in which to comply with these changes.

Exercising Your Right to Request an Accounting

If you do wish to make a request for an accounting, as is the case with respect to the exercising of most of the individual rights under HIPAA, you should start by reviewing the applicable covered entity's notice of privacy practices. That notice should describe the process to be used when requesting an accounting. Typically, you will be asked to write a letter requesting an amendment or to complete a form provided by the covered entity.

The covered entity must act on the request within 60 days. It can, however, obtain another 30 days to respond as long as it provides you with a written explanation of the delay.

All patients are entitled to receive one accounting per year without charge. If you wish to request more than one accounting from a particular covered entity, the entity may charge a reasonable cost-based fee. The covered entity must make you aware of the amount of the fee in advance. If you have a good reason why you need multiple accountings in a given year (for example, if you are a victim of identity theft), you may wish to try to obtain a fee waiver from the entity. HIPAA does not require that a covered entity grant a fee waiver, but depending upon the circumstances, some covered entities may elect to do so. It does not hurt to ask so if the fee is a concern, you should consider requesting a waiver.

Sample Document 2.4 contains a sample request for accounting form. Again, before using this or any other sample form, you should be sure to check with your provider to see if they have their own form that you should utilize.

Limitations on Accounting Rights

While the right to an accounting does establish an important right, the right is subject to a number of exceptions that dilute some of the power of the rule. First, covered entities have not been required to account for disclosures made for treatment, payment, or health care operations. As discussed, this has been changed under the HITECH Act, and covered entities with EHRs are to begin to account for disclosures made in connection with treatment, payment, and health care operations.

Covered entities are also not required to account for disclosures that you have authorized. This may not be of great significance to those patients who limit the number and scope of authorizations that they execute. If, however, you have signed one or more broadly crafted authorizations, this exception can amount to a sizeable loophole, effectively eliminating your ability to track those disclosures you have authorized.

The Impact of State Law

Depending upon where you reside, you may have greater accounting rights under your applicable state's laws. For example, certain states may require a covered entity to respond more promptly than as provided under HIPAA. In addition, other federal laws can impact your accounting rights. For example, if your records are held by the federal government, such as if you are a recipient of Medicare or U.S. Department of Veterans Affairs benefits, you will also have a right to an accounting under the Privacy Act of 1974. As with the other rights discussed in this chapter, when exercising your right to an accounting, make sure to review the covered entity's policies and procedures, as well as other federal laws, and applicable state law.

The Right to Privacy Notice[13]

Overview

The HIPAA Privacy Rule requires that each covered entity publish a notice that describes the entity's policies concerning PHI. This notice, known as the notice of privacy practices, is to describe how the entity implements the HIPAA Privacy Rule. Because the HIPAA Privacy Rule mandates the inclusion of particular provisions in privacy notices, all compliance notices will contain the same elements. Still, while it is true that many HIPAA Privacy

SAMPLE DOCUMENT 2.4: SAMPLE REQUEST FOR ACCOUNTING

Purpose: This form is for use to document the patient's request for an accounting of disclosures of his/her protected health information.

Section A: Patient Requesting Accounting
Name:
Address:
Telephone:
E-mail:
Social Security number (or other identifier):

You have the right to an accounting of certain disclosures that your health care provider made of your protected health information. Your health care provider does not have to account for the following disclosures made:

→ **for treatment, payment, or health care operations activities,**
→ **to you, to your personal representative, or pursuant to your authorization or permission,**
→ **as part of a limited data set,**
→ **for national security or intelligence purposes,**
→ **to law enforcement officials or correctional institutions, or**
→ **incidental disclosures permitted by HHS Privacy regulations.**

To exercise your right to request an accounting of disclosures regarding our use or disclosure of your protected health information, please complete Section B.

Section B: Requested Accounting of Disclosures

For what period of time are you requesting accounting? From: ___/__ /20__ to: _____ /___ /20__

Do you have any specific disclosures of protected health information that you are interested in? If so, please describe.

You are entitled to one free disclosure accounting every 12 months. Your health care provider will charge you $_____ for each additional accounting you request during the same 12-month period.

You may withdraw your request for additional accountings within five working days of the request if you determine you do not wish to pay the service charge.

Patient's Signature: Date: _____/___ /20__

If this request is by a personal representative on behalf of the individual, complete the following:

Personal representative's name:
Relationship to individual:
You Are Entitled to a Copy of this Request

Notices will look similar; each notice will be specific to the particular organization and, thus, to understand the policies and procedures of your covered entity and to exercise any of your individual rights, you must review the specific notice of privacy practices of your covered entity.

The Privacy Rule requires covered entities to make a good-faith effort to obtain an acknowledgment from each patient acknowledging receipt of the privacy notice. The acknowledgment requirement is widely misunderstood. The workers who staff your physician's office will likely assume that it is mandatory to obtain each patient's signature, which is incorrect. However, because the requirement is so widely misunderstood, it may be very difficult, if not impossible, to convince the receptionist or office manager at your doctor's office that you do not need to sign the form. Accordingly, it may not be worth battling over the need to sign the acknowledgment form. That said, you should review the acknowledgment form carefully before you sign it. Some physicians may bundle other forms with the HIPAA notice of privacy practices acknowledgment form. So, when signing the acknowledgment, first make sure that it is indeed all that you are signing. Without careful review, you may end up signing a disclosure, authorization, or another form that you may not have intended to sign.

In practice, you should be given a notice of privacy practices and acknowledgment form each time that you visit a new physician. For some health care providers, you will be provided with the same notice of privacy practices along with the same acknowledgment on each visit. Where this is done, it is not done because of any legal requirement incumbent upon the provider. Rather, it is likely that the provider is doing it this way because it is easier to get everyone to sign on to the form on every visit than it is to track who is visiting the doctor for the first time. Regardless of how your provider handles the process, make sure you review the notice and certainly review the acknowledgement before signing it. You have the right to take a copy of the notice home for further review. Depending on the size and sophistication of the health care provider, you may also be able to find the notice of privacy practices online on the Web site for the applicable provider. It will also be accessible in the office of the physician.

Health plans must also provide you with a notice of privacy practices. In most cases, your health plan will send you a copy of the notice in the mail. If you have not received it or misplaced it and wish to review a copy of the notice, check the plan's Web site or contact them for another copy.

Key Components of the Notice of Privacy Practices

You will find that most privacy notices are quite similar to one another. However, there may be some variations from one notice to another, especially with respect to any procedural requirements. This is important. Each covered entity's notice of privacy practices should describe the entity's procedures for exercising patient rights. To maximize the likelihood that your efforts to exercise your rights will be fruitful, make sure you follow the specified procedures identified in the applicable notice of privacy practices. In addition, you may observe fairly significant differences between notices from health care providers and notices from health insurers. In addition, differences in state laws may result in different notices from covered entities in different states. Sample Document 2.5 depicts a sample HIPAA notice of privacy practices.

There are some notable features to look for when reviewing a covered entity's notice of privacy practices, as further described below:

Uses and disclosures: One of the most notable aspects of the HIPAA privacy notice is its explanation of the covered entity's use and disclosure of your PHI. In addition to identifying categories of uses and disclosures of PHI, the notice of privacy practices must provide illustrative examples to help patients better understand the identified uses and disclosures. As noted, because of the requirements of the HIPAA Privacy Rule, the privacy notices of HIPAA covered entities will be quite similar to one another. However, the first time you review a notice, you may be quite taken aback by the length and breadth of the permitted uses and disclosures. There are some uses and disclosures that are particularly notable:

(i) **Fund-raising:** A health care provider may use your PHI in a limited way for fund-raising purposes. You have the right to opt out and tell the hospital not to use your records for fund-raising. If you say nothing, then the use of your records for fund-raising is permissible. Exercising this opt-out right may not be of critical importance, but it helps everyone if some people exercise opt-out rights when they exist. The HITECH Act is implementing some changes to the fund-raising rules, particularly with regard to disclosures about fundraising and opt-out rights. The rules concerning fund-raising will be discussed further in Chapter 6 regarding marketing activities involving health information.

(ii) **National security disclosures:** A covered entity can disclose your records for just about any national security purpose. The rule does not require a warrant, court order, subpoena, or any other procedures prior to the disclosure.

Your rights: The notice of privacy practices also outlines the individual rights that you have under HIPAA and that have been the primary focus of this chapter. In addition to outlining these various rights, the notice provides information about how to exercise those rights.

Contact information: Contact information for the covered entity's privacy officer will likely be found at the end of the notice. If you have any questions, want to exercise your rights, or wish to file a complaint with the covered entity, the privacy officer for the covered entity is probably the first person to contact.

SAMPLE DOCUMENT 2.5: NOTICE OF PRIVACY PRACTICES
NOTICE OF PRIVACY PRACTICES

Effective Date: _____

This notice describes how medical information about you may be used and disclosed and how you can get access to this information.

Please review it carefully.

If you have any questions about this notice, please contact _____.

Who Must Follow This Notice

This notice describes the privacy practices of (fill in a description of to whom or what entities the notice applies).

Our Obligations

We are required by law to:

• Maintain the privacy of protected health information;
• Give you this notice of our legal duties and privacy practices regarding health information about you; and
• Follow the terms of our notice that is currently in effect.

How We May Use And Disclose Health Information:

The following categories describe ways that we may use and disclose health information that identifies you ("Health Information"). Some of the categories include examples, but every type of use or disclosure of Health Information in a category is not listed. Except for the purposes described below, we will use and disclose Health Information only with your written permission. If you give us permission to use or disclose Health Information for a purpose not discussed in this notice, you may revoke that permission, in writing, at any time, by _____.

→ *For Treatment.* We may use Health Information to treat you or provide you with health care services. We may disclose Health Information to doctors, nurses, technicians, or other personnel, including people outside our facility who may be involved in your medical care. For example, we may tell your primary physician about the care we provided you or give your Health Information to a specialist to provide you with additional services.

→ *For Payment.* We may use and disclose Health Information so that we or others may bill or receive payment from you, an insurance company, or a third party for the treatment and services you received. For example, we may give them your health plan information about your treatment so that they will pay for such treatment. We also may tell your health plan about a treatment that you are going to receive to obtain prior approval or to determine whether your plan will cover it.

→ *For Health Care Operations.* We may use and disclose Health Information for health care operations purposes. These uses and disclosures are necessary to make sure that all of our patients receive quality care and for our operation and management purposes. For example, we may use your Health Information to review the treatment and services we provide to ensure that the care you receive is of the highest quality.

→ *Fund-Raising Activities.* We may use Health Information to contact you in an effort to raise money. We may disclose Health Information to a related foundation or to our business associate so that they may contact you to raise money for us.[1]

→ *Individuals Involved in Your Care or Payment for Your Care.* We may release your Health Information to a person who is involved in your medical care or helps pay for your care, such as a family member or friend. We also may notify your family about your location or general condition or disclose such information to an entity assisting in a disaster-relief effort.

→ *Research.* Under certain circumstances, we may use and disclose your Health Information for research purposes. For example, a research project may involve comparing the health and recovery of all patients who received one medication or treatment to those who received another, for the same condition. Before we use or disclose Health Information for research, though, the project will go through a special approval process. This process evaluates a proposed research project and its use of Health Information to balance the benefits of research with the need for privacy of Health Information. Even without special approval, we may permit researchers to look at records to help them identify patients who may be included in their research project or for other similar purposes, so long as they do not remove or take a copy of any Health Information.

Special Circumstances

→ *As Required by Law.* We will disclose Health Information when required to do so by international, federal, state, or local law.

→ *To Avert a Serious Threat to Health or Safety.* We may use and disclose Health Information when necessary to prevent or lessen a serious threat to your health and safety or the health and safety of the public or another person. Any disclosure, however, will be to someone who may be able to help prevent the threat.

→ *Business Associates.* We may disclose Health Information to our business associates who perform functions on our behalf or provide us with services if the information is necessary for such functions or services. For example, we may use another company to perform billing services on our behalf. All of our business associates are obligated, under contract with us, to protect the privacy of your information and are not allowed to use or disclose any information other than as specified in our contract.

→ *Organ and Tissue Donation.* If you are an organ donor, we may release Health Information to organizations that handle organ procurement or organ, eye, or tissue transplantation or to an organ donation bank, as necessary, to facilitate organ or tissue donation and transplantation.

→ *Military and Veterans*. If you are a member of the armed forces, we may release Health Information as required by military command authorities. We also may release Health Information to the appropriate foreign military authority if you are a member of a foreign military.

→ *Workers' Compensation*. We may release Health Information for workers' compensation or similar programs. These programs provide benefits for work-related injuries or illness.

→ *Public Health Risks*. We may disclose Health Information for public health activities. These activities generally include disclosures to prevent or control disease, injury, or disability; report births and deaths; report child abuse or neglect; report reactions to medications or problems with products; notify people of recalls of products they may be using; track certain products and monitor their use and effectiveness; notify a person who may have been exposed to a disease or may be at risk for contracting or spreading a disease or condition; and conduct medical surveillance of the office in certain limited circumstances concerning workplace illness or injury. We also may release Health Information to an appropriate government authority if we believe a patient has been the victim of abuse, neglect, or domestic violence; however, we will release this information only if you agree or when we are required or authorized by law.

→ *Health Oversight Activities*. We may disclose Health Information to a health oversight agency for activities authorized by law. These oversight activities include, for example, audits, investigations, inspections, and licensure. These activities are necessary for the government to monitor the health care system, government programs, and compliance with civil rights laws.

→ *Lawsuits and Disputes*. If you are involved in a lawsuit or a dispute, we may disclose Health Information in response to a court or administrative order. We also may disclose Health Information in response to a subpoena, discovery request, or other lawful process by someone else involved in the dispute, but only if efforts have been made to tell you about the request or to obtain an order protecting the information requested.

→ *Law Enforcement*. We may release Health Information if asked by a law enforcement official for the following reasons: (1) in response to a court order, subpoena, warrant, summons, or similar process; (2) limited information to identify or locate a suspect, fugitive, material witness, or missing person; (3) about the victim of a crime if, under certain limited circumstances, we are unable to obtain the person's agreement; (4) about a death we believe may be the result of criminal conduct; (5) about criminal conduct on our premises; and (6) in emergency circumstances to report a crime, the location of the crime or victims, or the identity, description, or location of the person who committed the crime.

→ ***Coroners, Medical Examiners, and Funeral Directors***. We may release Health Information to a coroner or medical examiner. This may be necessary, for example, to identify a deceased person or determine the cause of death. We also may release Health Information to funeral directors as necessary for their duties.

→ ***National Security and Intelligence Activities***. We may release Health Information to authorized federal officials for intelligence, counterintelligence, and other national security activities authorized by law.

→ ***Protective Services for the President and Others***. We may disclose Health Information to authorized federal officials so they may provide protection to the president, other authorized persons or foreign heads of state, or to conduct special investigations.

→ ***Inmates or Individuals in Custody***. If you are an inmate of a correctional institution or under the custody of a law enforcement official, we may release Health Information to the appropriate correctional institution or law enforcement official. This release would be made only if necessary (1) for the institution to provide you with health care; (2) to protect your health and safety or the health and safety of others; or (3) for the safety and security of the correctional institution.

Your Rights

You have the following rights regarding Health Information we maintain about you:

→ ***Right to Inspect and Copy***. You have the right to inspect and copy Health Information that may be used to make decisions about your care or payment for your care. To inspect and copy this Health Information, you must make your request in writing to _____.

→ ***Right to Amend***. If you feel that the Health Information we have is incorrect or incomplete, you may ask us to amend the information. You have the right to request an amendment for as long as the information is kept by or for us. To request an amendment, you must make your request in writing to _____.

→ ***Right to an Accounting of Disclosures***. You have the right to request an accounting of certain disclosures of Health Information we made. To request an accounting of disclosures, you must make your request in writing to _____.

→ ***Right to Request Restrictions***. You have the right to request a restriction or limitation on the Health Information we use or disclose for treatment, payment, or health care operations. In addition, you have the right to request a limit on the Health Information we disclose about you to someone who is involved in your care or the payment for your care, like a family member or friend. For example, you could ask that we not share information about your surgery with your spouse. To request a restriction, you must make your request, in writing, to _____. *We are not required to agree to your request*. If we agree, we will comply with your request unless we need to use the information in certain emergency treatment situations.

→ ***Right to Request Confidential Communications***. You have the right to request that we communicate with you about medical matters in a certain way or at a certain location. For example, you can ask that we contact you only by mail or at work. To request confidential communications, you must make your request in writing to _____. Your request must specify how or where you wish to be contacted. We will accommodate reasonable requests.

→ ***Right to a Paper Copy of This Notice***. You have the right to a paper copy of this notice. You may ask us to give you a copy of this notice at any time. Even if you have agreed to receive this notice electronically, you are still entitled to a paper copy of this notice.

You may obtain a copy of this notice at our Web site, http://www._____.
To obtain a paper copy of this notice, _____.

Changes To This Notice

We reserve the right to change this notice. We reserve the right to make the revised or changed notice effective for Health Information we already have, as well as any information we receive in the future. We will post a copy of the current notice at our office. The notice will contain the effective date on the first page in the top right-hand corner.

Complaints

If you believe your privacy rights have been violated, you may file a complaint with us or the Secretary of the Department of Health and Human Services. To file a complaint with us, contact _____. All complaints must be made in writing. You will not be penalized for filing a complaint.

[Name Of Company]

On ___ [date] _____. __ [Patient Name] _____ was given notice of the Privacy Practices of _____ [Name of Company] _____ by ___ [describe means by which you will provide notice to patients] _____.

Acknowledgement of Receipt Of Privacy Notice

I acknowledge that I was provided with a copy of the [name of company] notice of privacy practices.

_____   _____
Patient Signature   Date

[If you are unable to provide the notice of privacy practices to the patient because of an emergency treatment situation, describe below the good-faith efforts that you made to provide such notice to the patient after the emergency treatment situation was over.]

_____   _____

Name of Employee   **Date**

_____

[1]The HITECH Act is changing certain aspects of a covered entity's rights to use PHI for fund-raising purposes. These changes are discussed in further detail in Chapter 6 on health marketing.

The Right to Request Confidential Communications[14]

Overview

HIPAA also establishes the right to request confidential communications. This means that you have the right to request that your health care provider contact you by alternative means or at alternative locations. For example, you may not want your doctor to contact you at work or to leave certain messages on your home answering machine. Also, you may not want to receive a postcard reminder about the necessity of a follow-up visit from certain doctors. For instance, while you may find a postcard reminder of a dental cleaning appointment to be perfectly acceptable, you may not want to receive a reminder of a chemotherapy appointment to be sent in the same fashion. In this case, you may wish to request that your doctor contact you by sending the reminder in a closed envelope, as opposed to an open postcard that anyone could read.

The right to request confidential communications can be overlooked as not terribly significant but it is actually a very important right because a health provider does not need express permission to contact a patient at home or to leave a message on a home answering machine. Some providers will ask you where you wish to be contacted and where they can leave messages for you. However, not all providers will do this. The right is thus very important, especially for individuals who may not want their family to be aware of certain doctors they are seeing and/or certain medical treatments they are seeking.

Exercising Your Right to Request Confidential Communications

If you wish to receive confidential communications, you should submit a request to your health care provider. First, you should review your provider's notice of privacy practices to understand their required procedures. Some doctors may require you to make a formal written request for confidential communications. In a smaller office, an oral request may be sufficient. However, even where the provider informs you that an oral request is sufficient, you should consider making a written request. This may improve the likelihood that your request will be complied with, especially if there are personnel changes or temporary workers who may not be fully aware of the oral request that you had made. You should also take and retain a copy of the request that you submit to your provider.

The HIPAA Privacy Rule does not require the provider to respond to your request. Accordingly, it is very likely that you may not receive a confirmation of the request or any acknowledgment that the provider plans on complying with the request. You may, however, ask for a written acknowledgment. If the provider does respond to your request for an acknowledgment, you are well advised to retain that acknowledgment.

You do not have any obligation to explain your reason for making the request. In fact, the HIPAA Privacy Rule prohibits a health care provider from requiring you to provide an explanation as a condition of fulfilling the request. This is not to say that the provider is prohibited from asking you for a reason—the provider can ask, but you do not have to disclose the reason.

A health care provider is required to agree to a reasonable request for confidential communications. There is not a clear explanation as to what would constitute a reasonable request. However, it seems likely that a request to contact you at your office phone instead of your home phone would be reasonable. It also seems likely that a request to receive all appointment reminders via FedEx may not be considered reasonable.

Health plans also need to honor requests for confidential communications, but there are some important distinctions. With respect to requests for confidential communications that are made to health plans, the individual must clearly state that the disclosure of all or part of the information could endanger the patient. The health plan may require that a request contain a statement that disclosure could endanger the patient.

Even if the covered entity agrees to your request for confidential communications, there is an exception for emergencies. This means that in the event of an emergency, such as a need to provide emergency treatment to you, the covered entity may ignore the restrictions it may have previously agreed upon with you.

The Right to Request Restrictions on Uses or Disclosures of PHI[15]

Overview

Under the HIPAA Privacy Rule, a covered entity must allow an individual to request a restriction on the use or disclosure of his or her information in order to carry out treatment, payment, or health care operations. In addition, the covered entity must also permit a patient to request restrictions on disclosures of PHI to family members, relatives, or close friends. It is extremely important to emphasize that this "right" merely allows an individual to request these restrictions; it does not require a covered entity to comply with the individual's request, not even where the request is reasonable. Thus, this "right" is quite distinct from the right to request confidential communications discussed in the previous section. You may recall that covered entities must comply with requests for confidential communications, provided that such requests are reasonable. Regarding restrictions, however, a covered entity need not even respond to a request for restrictions. The value of this "right" is thus truly questionable.

Even worse, under HIPAA, some restrictions that an institution might agree to will not even be effective. These are uses or disclosures that are permitted for facility directories (separate rules govern facility directories), to HHS for oversight of HIPAA, or for any of the scores of other permissible disclosures allowed under HIPAA.

The HITECH Act has modified this right in a limited way. Specifically, the HITECH Act requires a covered entity to agree to a requested restriction if the disclosure is to a health plan for the purposes of payment or health care operations and the PHI pertains to an item or service for which the health care provider has been paid in full. Essentially, this means that the HITECH Act reimburses individuals who pay for an item or service out of pocket in full with a means of restricting access to their PHI by health plans. This could be a fairly important right for patients who may be interested in keeping certain treatments, diagnoses, or other information from being shared with their health insurer.

How to Exercise Your Right to Request Restrictions

In practice, it is likely to be extremely difficult to convince many covered entities to agree to any restrictions on uses or disclosures. It is possible that a small practice may agree to certain reasonable requests, but it is unlikely that a large provider will agree to honor such a request.

You may have more luck in getting a health care provider to agree to limit disclosures to relatives and friends. If you tell your doctor or nurse not to talk to a relative, that provider is likely to comply. In practice, however, it may be quite difficult to obtain or enforce a formal agreement.

If you are dealing with your family doctor in a smaller office and ask her, verbally, to please ensure that your diagnosis is not shared with your spouse or children, she will likely comply with that request. However, getting a written agreement may be more difficult or even impossible. The formality of the rule allows providers to insist that patients make requests in writing, and most will demand a letter.

Even if you do make a written request, HIPAA does not require the provider to respond to your request in a reasonable amount of time, or even to respond at all. Now, consider how this might play out in the case of hospitalization. Say, for example, you did not want a visiting family member to have certain details of your medical condition. In most cases, you would probably be treated and released before your formal request to limit disclosures was even received, let alone addressed.

The Right to Complain[16]

Complaint Process

HIPAA does not provide for an individual right of action, meaning aggrieved individuals are not able to sue medical providers, health insurance companies, and other covered entities for violating their privacy under HIPAA. However, individuals do have the right to complain about privacy practices to the covered entity and to the Secretary of HHS. Any person who believes that a covered entity is not complying with the HIPAA privacy rule may file a complaint with the Office of Civil Rights at the Department of Health and Human Services (OCR). One does not have to be a patient of a health care provider or a beneficiary of a health insurance plan to file a complaint. For example, if you visit a relative in the hospital and see a violation, you can file a complaint.

How to File a Complaint

If you wish to file a complaint for a HIPAA violation, you must take care to ensure that your complaint complies with certain procedural requirements. Your complaint must be filed in writing, either on paper or electronically, by mail, fax, or e-mail. It must name the health care or social service provider involved and it must describe the acts or omissions that you believed violated the civil rights laws or regulations. You can use the complaint form at http://www.hhs.gov/ocr/privacy/hipaa/complaints/howtofileahealthinformationprivacycomplaintpkg.pdf or at http://www.hhs.gov/ocr/privacy/hipaa/complaints/index.html. You can submit a complaint online to OCRComplaint@hhs.gov.

Complaints must be filed within 180 days of when you knew that the act or omission complained of occurred. OCR may extend the 180-day period if you can show "good cause" for the delay. If you mail or fax the complaint, be sure to send it to the appropriate OCR regional office based on where the alleged violation took place. OCR has 10 regional offices, and each regional office covers specific states. Send your complaint to the attention of the OCR regional manager.

You can find a fact sheet on the complaint process at http://www.hhs.gov/ocr/privacy/hipaa/complaints/index.html. The fact sheet lists addresses of the regional offices of the Office of Civil Rights that will accept your complaint.

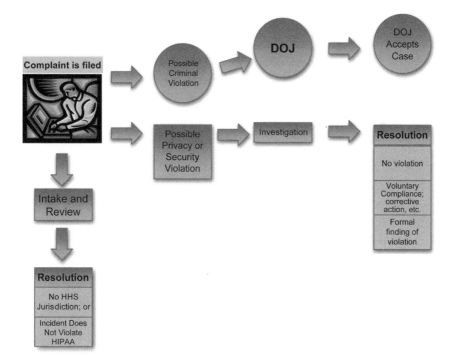

Figure 2.1   The Complaint Process

This information is also included below in Table 2.1. The government also operates a toll free telephone number for help with complaints. The number is 1-800-368-1019.

Under Civil Rights Laws, an entity cannot retaliate against you for filing a complaint. You should notify OCR immediately in the event of any retaliatory action.

BEYOND COMPLAINTS

There are valid reasons for questioning the value of filing a complaint with OCR. After all, OCR does not have a strong track record of pursuing enforcement actions against those covered entities on which complaints have been filed. This may be changing under the Obama Administration, which has already adopted a pro-privacy approach in a number of areas. With the fines and penalties for HIPAA violations being increased under the HITECH Act, it does seem likely that enforcement will be stepped up. Accordingly, if you are aware of a violation, you should consider filing a complaint with OCR.

You should also consider complaining directly to the applicable covered entity. All covered entities must have a HIPAA Privacy Officer. The name, address, and telephone number should be included in the covered entity's

TABLE 2.1
OCR: Regional Office Addresses

Region I: Boston (Connecticut, Maine, Massachusetts, New Hampshire, Rhode Island, Vermont)

Peter Chan, Regional Manager
Office for Civil Rights
U.S. Department of Health and Human Services
Government Center
J.F. Kennedy Federal Building, Room 1875
Boston, MA 02203
Voice phone (617) 565-1340
Fax (617) 565-3809
TDD (617) 565-1343

Region II: New York (New Jersey, New York, Puerto Rico, Virgin Islands)

Michael Carter, Regional Manager
Office for Civil Rights
U.S. Department of Health and Human Services
Jacob Javits Federal Building
26 Federal Plaza, Suite 3312
New York, NY 10278
Voice Phone (212) 264-3313
Fax (212) 264-3039
TDD (212) 264-2355

Region III: Philadelphia (Delaware, District of Columbia, Maryland, Pennsylvania, Virginia, West Virginia)

Paul Cushing, Regional Manager
Office for Civil Rights
U.S. Department of Health and Human Services
150 S. Independence Mall West
Suite 372, Public Ledger Building
Philadelphia, PA 19106-9111
Main Line (215) 861-4441
Hotline (800) 368-1019
Fax (215) 861-4431
TDD (215) 861-4440

Region IV: Atlanta (Alabama, Florida, Georgia, Kentucky, Mississippi, North Carolina, South Carolina, Tennessee)

Roosevelt Freeman, Regional Manager
Office for Civil Rights

(Continued)

TABLE 2.1 (*Continued*)

U.S. Department of Health and Human Services

Atlanta Federal Center, Suite 3B70

61 Forsyth Street, S.W.

Atlanta, GA 30303-8909

Voice Phone (404) 562-7886

Fax (404) 562-7881

TDD (404) 331-2867

Region V: Chicago (Illinois, Indiana, Michigan, Minnesota, Ohio, Wisconsin)

Valerie Morgan-Alston, Regional Manager

Office for Civil Rights

U.S. Department of Health and Human Services

233 N. Michigan Ave., Suite 240

Chicago, IL 60601

Voice Phone (312) 886-2359

Fax (312) 886-1807

TDD (312) 353-5693

Region VI: Dallas (Arkansas, Louisiana, New Mexico, Oklahoma, Texas)

Ralph Rouse, Regional Manager

Office for Civil Rights

U.S. Department of Health and Human Services

1301 Young Street, Suite 1169

Dallas, TX 75202

Voice Phone (214) 767-4056

Fax (214) 767-0432

TDD (214) 767-8940

Region VII: Kansas City (Iowa, Kansas, Missouri, Nebraska)

Frank Campbell, Regional Manager

Office for Civil Rights

U.S. Department of Health and Human Services

601 East 12th Street, Room 248

Kansas City, MO 64106

Voice Phone (816) 426-7277

Fax (816) 426-3686

TDD (816) 426-7065

(*Continued*)

TABLE 2.1   (*Continued*)

Region VIII: Denver (Colorado, Montana, North Dakota, South Dakota, Utah, Wyoming)

Velveta Howell, Regional Manager
Office for Civil Rights
U.S. Department of Health and Human Services
1961 Stout Street, Room 1426 FOB
Denver, CO 80294-3538
Voice Phone (303) 844-2024
Fax (303) 844-2025
TDD (303) 844-3439

Region IX: San Francisco (American Samoa, Arizona, California, Guam, Hawaii, Nevada)

Michael Kruley, Regional Manager
Office for Civil Rights
U.S. Department of Health and Human Services
90 7th Street, Suite 4-100
San Francisco, CA 94103
Voice Phone (415) 437-8310
Fax (415) 437-8329
TDD (415) 437-8311

Region X: Seattle(Alaska, Idaho, Oregon, Washington)

Linda Yuu Connor, Regional Manager
Office for Civil Rights
U.S. Department of Health and Human Services
2201 Sixth Avenue, M/S: RX-11
Seattle, WA 98121-1831
Voice Phone (206) 615-2290
Fax (206) 615-2297
TDD (206) 615-2296

---

notice of privacy practices. The covered entity may not be aware of the incident that gave rise to your wish to file a complaint. Receiving your complaint will provide the covered entity with the information needed to investigate the problem and, hopefully, make things right.

In any case, when making a complaint, you should think carefully about the possible ramifications. As noted above, HIPAA prohibits OCR from retaliating against people who file complaints. However, filing a complaint may bring more attention to you and the health information that you are seeking to keep private. Accordingly, you may wish to be careful about disclosing significant PHI in your medical record. You can also request confidential treatment in your complaint, and some authorities may be willing to grant your request.

Filing a complaint for a HIPAA violation may not rectify your problem nor result in a change in the practices of the applicable covered entity. However, by complaining, you are educating others about situations that you feel violate your privacy. You are also alerting lawmakers about deficiencies in health privacy law. You are not likely to see changes overnight, but if enough people communicate their dissatisfaction, we might see improvements in the future.

If your complaints to the OCR and/or the applicable covered entity prove ineffective, you may consider other courses of action. For example, you might be able to complain to a state official. Every state has a health department and an insurance department. In addition, health care providers hold licenses from state boards. If the violation is serious, see if the state licensing board accepts public complaints.

You may also wish to contact your state's attorney general. As noted, the changes to HIPAA that have been ushered in by the HITECH Act authorize state attorneys general to bring actions for HIPAA violations. Attorneys general are likely to flex their newly affirmed rights to bring enforcement actions under HIPAA. In fact, the first such action has already been filed—and settled. In early 2010, Connecticut Attorney General (AG) Richard Blumenthal became the first state attorney general to bring suit for a HIPAA violation when he filed a claim against Health Net of Connecticut, Inc. (HealthNet). The legal action arose out of the disappearance of a portable drive from the company's premises in Connecticut. Reportedly, the lost or stolen drive contained PHI and other data on more than 1.5 million current and former members of HealthNet.[17] The lawsuit, which claimed that HealthNet violated HIPAA, sought injunctive relief and statutory damages. With regard to the sought-after injunctive relief, AG Blumenthal had sought a court order that would block HealthNet from continued violations of HIPAA by requiring that it encrypt any PHI stored on any portable devices. The case was recently settled after HealthNet agreed to pay $250,000 to settle the suit.[18] Under the terms of the settlement, HealthNet will also provide those who were impacted by the breach with two years of credit monitoring services, $1 million of identity theft insurance and reimbursement for the cost of security freezes.

In some cases, you may also wish to contact the media. If your problem is newsworthy and you are willing to make it public, you might look for a local reporter who covers health issues and who may be interested in your story. However, it will be essential to exercise a lot of caution here. While going public with your story may help to bring a lot of attention to the covered entity

Fling a Complaint With Your State:

If you do wish to pursue a complaint with your state's attorney general, you should first investigate whether your state has implemented a formalized procedures for receiving complaints. Some states have consumer complaint forms that are designed specifically for healthcare-related complaints. The table below contains links to a number of forms for filing consumer complaints. Remember that the right of state attorneys general to file HIPAA complaints is relatively new. Accordingly, many states do not have specific HIPAA-oriented complaint forms. If you do not find a form for your state here, check the web site for your state's attorney general or contact them by phone to inquire as to how to file your complaint.

Arizona	http://www.azag.gov/AllComplaints.html
Connecticut	http://www.ct.gov/ag/lib/ag/health/complaintform.pdf
Georgia	http://www.georgia.gov/00/channel_title/ 0,2094,4802_5041,00.html
Maine	http://www.maine.gov/ag/consumer/complaints/index. shtml
Michigan	http://www.michigan.gov/ag/0,1607,7-164-17331---,00.html
Nevada	http://ag.state.nv.us/complaints/complaints.htm
New Hampshire	http://doj.nh.gov/consumer/complaints.html
New York	http://www.ag.ny.gov/bureaus/health_care/pdfs/complaint_ form.pdf
Ohio	http://www.ohioattorneygeneral.gov/ConsumerComplaint
Pennsylvania	http://www.attorneygeneral.gov/uploadedFiles/Complaints/ healthcare.pdf
Texas	http://www.oag.state.tx.us/consumer/complain.shtml
Virginia	http://www.vdacs.virginia.gov/forms-pdf/cp/oca/complaint/ oca1complaint.pdf
West Virginia	http://www.wvago.gov/publications.cfm

that has violated your privacy rights, it will also bring a lot of attention to your health information and may thus make your privacy violations worse.

As noted, HIPAA does not include a private right of action, meaning it does not provide patients with the right to sue covered entities. However, depending upon the nature of the violation giving rise to your complaint, you may be empowered to sue under other laws. For example, a violation of HIPAA may also constitute a violation of state law under which a lawsuit can be filed. Lawsuits can be very expensive and highly time-consuming. In addition, they may not achieve the results you desire. Accordingly, for many privacy violations, lawsuits may not be the best answer.

CONCLUSION

This chapter has delved into the individual rights that are afforded to you under HIPAA and has explained how those rights may be exercised. While it is true that there are a number of justifiable complaints that can be levied against HIPAA, it is also undeniable that it does convey a number of important rights and has made important strides in protecting medical privacy. All too often, individuals are not aware of the scope of their rights and are unsure as to how they may exercise those rights. This chapter has endeavored to elucidate these important points in the hope that it may empower individuals to assume a more active role in the protection of their own health information privacy.

Next up, in Chapter 3, we will examine the threats to the security of your medical information. It will focus upon the various threats to medical information privacy and security, such as lost and stolen laptops, unauthorized access to information, and medical identity theft. It will also examine the legal requirements that are applicable to the entities that collect, use, and disclose your medical information. Finally, it will examine the steps that you can and should take to reduce the likelihood that the security of your medical information may be compromised.

3

Data Insecurity, Breaches, and ID Theft

INTRODUCTION

Understanding the Risks

The security of medical information is a major issue that must be an integral part of any discussion concerning health privacy. Continued technological advances and more widespread use of technology are resulting in PHI being distributed through more channels than ever before, and as more medical providers and insurers transition to electronic health records, the potential risks to the security of health information may continue to grow. While it is true that technology can help to protect the security of data, it can also create new risks, many of which are due to the fact that technology can make information more compact, more easily transportable and transferable, and more easy to access. Of course, the security of medical information also remains vulnerable to old threats, including improperly discarded documents and lost papers.

Consider the following examples that aim to illustrate just how easily the privacy and security of medical information can be placed at risk:

Taking your dog for a walk one breezy evening, you are troubled by large amounts of small receipts and other papers scattered along the ground. As your pup, Toby, is preoccupied sniffing around a tree, you begin to collect some of this litter in order to throw it in the trash. As you gather up the papers, you observe the logo of your local pharmacy. You make a mental note of this, intending to complain about the mess to the pharmacy in the morning. As you look more closely at the papers you are gathering, however, you see that many of them contain individual patient names and addresses, as well as their prescription names, diagnoses, insurance information, and billing information.

Your little sister, Anne, calls you in tears, screaming and crying that her life has been ruined. Anne sought medical care at a health clinic where she was diagnosed with a sexually transmitted disease. Laura, an ex-girlfriend of Anne's current boyfriend, Tim, was a file clerk at the clinic and, after seeing Anne in the waiting room, pulled her file to satisfy her curiosity about key details about Anne, such as her weight. Upon reviewing the file, Laura reads the doctors, notes about Anne's diagnosis and feels as if she has struck gold. Rapidly, she grabs her phone and captures a photo of the diagnosis sheet, which she immediately sends via text message to 30 of her closest friends. Some of these friends forward the image on to other friends and many post it online to various social-networking sites. Anne tells you she is now the subject of relentless teasing and taunting. She says she can never return to school and says she wants to kill herself.

Susan, a claims processor at a medical center, is completely overworked and cannot seem to manage to get through her workload. As a result, she ends up bringing home extra work each night. Last night, exhausted, she fell asleep on the train on the way home. While she was sleeping, someone grabbed her backpack containing her laptop. That laptop contained a wide range of patient information, including names, addresses, medical conditions, Social Security numbers, recent payments, payment methods, and contact information. The information was password-protected but not encrypted. After Susan got off at her stop, Alan, her seatmate, noticed the laptop. He was about to the alert the conductor, but then, thinking about his tight finances, thought that he may be able to make some money off of the laptop. So Alan grabbed the laptop and took it with him when he got off at the next step. He sold the laptop—and the data stored on it—and it eventually ended up in the hands of identity thieves.

TakeControl is an online resource where individuals can compile, maintain, access, and share their personal health records. One of TakeControl's main selling points has been its ultra-high security. The company was founded by a team of medical doctors and former high-level security officials from the U.S. government. However, despite the expertise of the team, the Web site was left vulnerable to attack by a well-known programming weakness, and two days ago, a hacker intruded into the Web site, taking a wide range of consumers' health data, which it is presently analyzing and mining with the goal of selling it for the highest price.

While startling and troubling, unfortunately, these examples are not mere hypothetical cases. Rather, they are based upon the facts of actual cases. As technology has made our lives easier in so many ways, it has also helped to increase the vulnerability of the privacy and security of our medical information. Consider, for example, the second vignette above. Prior to the advent of text messaging and online social networking, Laura may have had to call her friends to spread this nasty bit of gossip. Sure, this still would have spread the news about Anne, but the process would have taken more time. Additionally, her friends may have found the rumor less credible without seeing the actual medical report that Laura had sent via text message. Of course, Laura could have also made copies of the report and mailed them to a bunch of people, perhaps even posted them around the school and the shopping mall, but none of these other options would have the same instantaneous and widespread effect as the impact Laura was able to make with her cell phone and social-networking account.

The risk to the security of personal information goes far beyond online concerns, however. Medical information is vulnerable to a vast number of security risks, some of which are identified in the summary below.

The Importance of Information Security

Security and privacy are closely interrelated and completely interdependent. A health care provider may have very strict privacy policies that prohibit data access and use in all but a few clearly defined circumstances. However, if that provider fails to implement sufficient technical, administrative, and organizational measures to ensure that these policies are maintained, they will have very little value at all. Likewise, an organization can have a very protective security program in place, but these security measures will be of relatively little value if that organization's privacy policies and procedures permit liberal data access and use.

The main goals of information security are to ensure that: (1) only authorized individuals can access certain data; (2) authorized individuals can access the data only when they need to use it for an authorized purpose; and (3) the data that authorized individuals can access is accurate. Traditionally, these goals have been pursued through various protections that are intended to ensure that data is safe from unauthorized access, alteration, deletion, or transmission.

TABLE 3.1
Common Risks to Medical Security

- Hospital staff leaving medical notes unattended at a public counter
- Health care providers' failing to dispose of health records in a secure manner
- Inadequate controls regarding which staff can access health information
- Storing sensitive data on a laptop computer that is taken off-site and not stored securely
- A pharmacist discussing a consumer's medications and medical conditions with her in a manner that is audible to others
- A health insurance company's failure to train its employees about the importance of information security

The vigorous pursuit of these goals in the face of new threats is essential. As outlined in the Introduction, unauthorized access to medical information can have a number of extremely negative consequences. In addition to embarrassment, possible discrimination, and numerous other consequences to the individual whose information has been breached, the failure to protect the security of medical information can result in medical identity theft, which, in turn, can result not only in significant financial consequences, but can also jeopardize the health and very lives of its victims.[1] In cases of medical ID theft, someone without medical insurance who needs surgery, medical treatment, or prescription drugs will steal someone's medical identity in order to utilize the insurance of the victim and obtain the necessary care. The victim is left with bills for unpaid claims and, potentially, erroneous medical information in their records. Reversing the effects of medical ID theft can be very difficult as there is no straightforward, centralized process for challenging false medical claims or correcting inaccurate medical records. For years after falling victim to identity theft, an individual can be left with large amounts of unpaid bills, a tarnished credit report, and inaccurate medical records, not to mention high levels of stress and aggravation, all with little recourse.

What to Expect from this Chapter

This chapter will commence with a review of the legal framework applicable to data security. It will provide details on the data security obligations of the Health Insurance Portability and Accountability Act (HIPAA).[2] It will also call into question the efficacy of these legal measures by showing how private health information still remains vulnerable to breaches, theft, and unauthorized access. This chapter also examines one of the most serious consequences of data insecurity: medical identity theft. By exploring case studies, this chapter will demonstrate the risks of medical identity theft and offer clear tips and strategies for protecting yourself against this very dangerous practice.

A BRIEF REVIEW OF DATA SECURITY LAW

Overview

Recently, lawmakers and regulators have begun to place a lot of emphasis on data security. In the not-so-distant past, lawmakers had been emphasizing privacy requirements and, in some cases, data security was a small part of more generalized privacy laws. However, more recently, data security has emerged as an area of particular emphasis. This new focus on data security is with good cause, as without proper security, the privacy and confidentiality of medical information cannot be assured. Public perceptions about data security issues may also be influencing the attention that lawmakers are directing to new laws to protect information. A recent Harris poll, for example, concluded that millions of Americans believe that their medical records have been compromised.[3]

Are these fears unfounded or blown out of proportion? Not according to recent data. It seems that virtually every day there are new stories of lost laptops, stolen files, and other unauthorized acts that compromise the security and integrity of medical information. Recent data from California exemplifies this very point. Since January 1, 2009, health care organizations in California have been required to notify regulators in the event of a breach involving health information. In the several months since that law entered into force, organizations have reported more than 800 data breaches involving medical information.[4] This figure, large by any estimation, is truly astounding when one considers that this number concerns only one state and only a six-month time period. In addition in the six-month period between September 22, 2009, and February 2, 2010 (the first period of time in which HHS posted this breach list to its site), over 40 breaches, each impacting more than 500 people, were reported.[5]

As the following sections will show, covered entities, business associates, and other companies with access to medical information are subject to a number of laws that require them to protect the security of the medical information within their possession. The next section will examine the current legal framework, which imposes a number of data security obligations on entities that collect, use, and/or disclose medical information. While the HIPAA Security Rule is among the most significant of these laws, as will be discussed, there are other legal requirements that mandate the implementation of specific data security measures to protect medical information.

The HIPAA Security Rule

General Principles

As outlined in the Introduction and Chapter 1, HIPAA is comprehensive legislation that aims to achieve a number of goals. Most relevant to the topic of this chapter is the HIPAA Security Rule, which specifies a series of administrative, technical, and physical security procedures that must be implemented to protect the confidentiality and security of electronic protected health information (ePHI or electronic PHI). Before HIPAA, there were no established security requirements or even generally accepted security standards. As such, despite the criticisms that can be made against the HIPAA Security Rule for not going far enough to protect data (e.g., it only applies to electronic PHI, enforcement has been relatively lax, etc.), it is also clear that the rule was an important development in information security.

An important distinction between the HIPAA Privacy Rule and the HIPAA Security Rule is that while the HIPAA Privacy Rule applies to all PHI (whether electronic, written, or oral), the HIPAA Security Rule only covers PHI that is in electronic form.[6] It does not apply to PHI that is stored on paper or disclosed verbally.

Under the HIPAA Security Rule, covered entities (and, more recently, by virtue of the HITECH Act, business associates) must:

- Ensure the confidentiality, integrity, and availability of ePHI that it creates, receives, maintains, or transmits;[7]

- Protect against any reasonably anticipated threats and hazards to the security or integrity of electronic PHI;[8] and

- Protect against reasonably anticipated uses or disclosures of such information that are not permitted by the HIPAA Privacy Rule.[9]

The HIPAA Security Rule requires that covered entities (and, now, business associates) implement data security standards in the following three areas:

- **Administrative safeguards**: Generally, these are administrative functions that should be implemented to meet the security standards.[10] An example of an administrative safeguard is "Security Awareness and Training." Entities are required to ensure that their workforce is made aware of their security obligations and receive adequate training.[11]

- **Physical safeguards**: Generally, these are the mechanisms that are required to protect the systems, equipment, and electronic data that is stored on them from threats, intrusions, and disasters.[12] Physical safeguards include, by way of example, media disposal practices, procedures for physical access to facilities in which systems are accessible and data back-up controls.

- **Technical safeguards**: These safeguards generally cover the technical processes that are used to protect and control access to PHI.[13] As an example, technical safeguards address the policies and procedures that are to be implemented to ensure the security of electronic transmissions, including transmissions sent via the Internet.

Within the three categories of administrative, physical, and technical safeguards are 18 standards. Twelve of these standards have implementation specifications. A standard defines what a covered entity must do, and implementation specifications describe how it must be done. The Security Rule has a total of 36 implementation specifications. The implementation specifications are further divided into two types: required (of which there are 14) and addressable (of which there are 22). Required specifications are critical, and covered entities must implement them as they are written. Addressable does not mean optional, but covered entities do have some options as to how the specifications are implemented. If a particular addressable implementation specification is determined to be reasonable and appropriate, the covered entity must implement it.[14] If a specific addressable implementation specification is not reasonable and appropriate, but the overall standard cannot be met without an additional security measure, a covered entity must (i) document why it would not be reasonable and appropriate to implement the implementation specification, and (ii) implement and document the alternative security measure that accomplishes the same purpose as the addressable implementation specification.[15] If implementing a specific addressable implementation specification is not reasonable and appropriate, but the overall standard can be met without implementation of an alternative security measure, a covered entity must document (i) the decision not to implement the addressable specification; (ii) why it would not be reasonable and appropriate to implement the implementation specification; and (iii) how the standard is being met.

Administrative Safeguards[16]

Administrative safeguards require documented policies and procedures for managing day-to-day operations, the conduct and access of workforce members to electronic PHI, and the selection, development, and use of security controls. The specific standards of the administrative safeguards are described below:

TABLE 3.2
Administrative Safeguards

Security-Management Process	An overall requirement to implement policies and procedures to prevent, detect, contain, and correct security violations.
Assigned Security Responsibility	A single individual must be designated as having overall responsibility for the security of a covered entity's electronic PHI.
Workforce Security	Policies, procedures, and processes must be developed and implemented to ensure that only properly authorized workforce members have access to electronic PHI.
Information Access Management	Policies, procedures, and processes must be developed and implemented for authorizing, establishing, and modifying access to electronic PHI.
Security Awareness and Training	A security awareness and training program for a covered entity's entire workforce must be developed and implemented.
Security Incident Procedures	Policies, procedures, and processes must be developed and implemented for reporting, responding to, and managing security incidents.

(Continued)

TABLE 3.2 (*Continued*)

Contingency Plan	Policies, procedures, and processes must be developed and implemented for responding to a disaster or emergency that damages information systems containing electronic PHI.
Evaluation	Covered entities must perform periodic technical and non-technical evaluations that determine the extent to which a covered entity's security policies, procedures, and processes meet the ongoing requirements of the HIPAA Security Rule.
Business Associate Contracts and other Arrangements	When dealing with business associates that create, receive, maintain, or transmit electronic PHI on the covered entity's behalf, the covered entity must develop and implement contracts that ensure the business associate will appropriately safeguard the information.

Physical Safeguards[17]

Physical safeguards are a series of requirements meant to protect a covered entity's electronic information systems and electronic PHI from unauthorized physical access. Covered entities must limit physical access while permitting properly authorized access. The specific standards are described in the chart that follows.

Technical Safeguards[18]

Technical safeguards are several requirements for using technology to protect electronic PHI, particularly controlling access to it. The specific standards are summarized in tables 3.3 and 3.4.

Enforcement of the HIPAA Security Rule

The Office of Civil Rights (OCR) now has responsibility for enforcing the HIPAA Security Rule. This is due to a shift announced July 27, 2009.[19] Previously, the Centers for Medicaid and Medicare Services (CMS) had responsibility for enforcing the HIPAA Security Rule and OCR had enforced only the HIPAA Privacy Rule. While it is too soon to tell, OCR may be well suited for enforcing the HIPAA Security Rule. Given well-established links between privacy and security, there has not been a clear rationale for the existence of two separate enforcement bodies, where one deals with privacy and the other deals with security. In addition, OCR has been a bit more visible

TABLE 3.3
Technical Safeguards

Facility Access Controls	An overall requirement to implement policies, procedures, and processes that limit physical access to electronic information systems while ensuring that properly authorized access is allowed.
Workstation Use	Policies and procedures must be developed and implemented that specify appropriate use of workstations and the characteristics of the physical environment of workstations that can access electronic PHI.
Workstation Security	Covered entities must implement physical safeguards for all workstations that can access electronic PHI in order to limit access to only authorized users.
Device and media controls	Policies, procedures, and processes must be developed and implemented for the receipt and removal of hardware and electronic media that contain electronic PHI into and out of a covered entity, and the movement of those items within a covered entity.

on the enforcement front and may have better infrastructure for investigating complaints and enforcing the requirements of HIPAA.

Data Breach Response Requirements

The high incidence of data breaches is a major threat to medical privacy and security. One way that lawmakers are attempting to mitigate the consequences of data breaches is by requiring organizations to notify individuals when their information has been subject to a breach or unauthorized access. These requirements are based upon the theory that if individuals are aware that their information has been compromised, they may be better prepared to watch out for any evidence that their information has been subject to unauthorized access. In addition to requirements found in state law, the HITECH Act has also introduced federal notification obligations for certain breaches involving PHI.

The HITECH Act

The breach notifications requirements established by the HITECH Act apply to HIPAA covered entities and business associates, as well as to PHR vendors and their service providers. The breach-notification obligations of the HITECH Act apply to a broad class of information. However, critically, the breach-no-

TABLE 3.4
Technical Safeguards

Access Controls	Policies, procedures, and processes must be developed and implemented for electronic information systems that contain electronic PHI to only allow access to persons or software programs that have appropriate access rights.
Audit Controls	Mechanisms must be implemented to record and examine activity in information systems that contain or use electronic PHI.
Integrity	Policies, procedures, and processes must be developed and implemented that protect electronic PHI from improper modification or destruction.
Person or Entity Authentication	Policies, procedures, and processes must be developed and implemented that verify that persons or entities seeking access to electronic PHI are who or what they claim to be.
Transmission Security	Policies, procedures, and processes must be developed and implemented that prevent unauthorized access to ePHI that is being transmitted over an electronic communications network.

tification obligation applies only when information is "unsecured." The term "unsecured protected health information" in the new notice provisions means:

[P]rotected health information that is not secured through the use of a technology or methodology specified by the Secretary . . . [and] protected health information that is not secured by a technology standard that renders protected health information unusable, unreadable, or indecipherable to unauthorized individuals and is developed or endorsed by a standards developing organization that is accredited by the American National Standards Institute[20]

HHS's implementing regulations (discussed further below under the HHS Rule) confirm that the idea of "secured" information includes both (i) "encrypted" information meeting certain technical standards and (ii) "destroyed" information. This exception should motivate companies to pursue new and expanded means of encrypting their customer information.

There are a few other limited exceptions to the broad breach-notification obligations. As one example, the statute creates an exception where the unauthorized recipient "would not reasonably have been able to retain the information."[21] One might imagine that this exception might apply, for example, when an individual had quick, limited access to a spreadsheet of PHI.

While the HITECH Act established the general rules applicable to data breach responses, further specificity is found in the rules promulgated under the HITECH Act. First, the HITECH Act required HHS to adopt a specific rule for HIPAA-covered entities and their business associates, defining and explaining the requirements related to breach notification. Second, it also required the FTC to promulgate a breach-notification rule for vendors of PHRs, many of whom are not otherwise covered by HIPAA. Those rules are discussed in the following sections.

The FTC Rule

The FTC, issuing its regulation (FTC Rule) on August 17, 2009,[22] focuses on two kinds of entities: (1) vendors of personal health records (companies that provide online repositories that people can use to keep track of their health information) and (2) entities that offer third-party applications for personal health records (the FTC's examples include devices such as blood pressure cuffs or pedometers that produce readings consumers can upload into their personal health records).

Much of the FTC Rule addresses issues of jurisdiction. In the FTC Rule, the FTC makes clear that its focus is on companies that are outside of HIPAA coverage. In fact, the FTC rule clarifies that (with very limited exceptions) the FTC's jurisdiction extends only to entities that are not subject to HHS jurisdiction, so that companies face only one regulator for these issues and consumers will receive only one notice in the event of a security breach.

The FTC Rule applies only to a limited class of entities, namely PHR vendors and companies that offer third party applications for PHRs. While advocates of greater regulation of health privacy may have been disappointed that the PHR vendors were not subject to more stringent privacy and/or data security requirements in the new legislation, this breach-notification rule represents the first step in the regulation of these entities, along with a future study requiring the FTC and HHS to consider a broader set of restrictions on their activities.

In its comments accompanying the rule, the FTC acknowledged the potential confusion arising from state security breach-notification laws, but made no effort to preempt these laws. Accordingly, entities covered by the FTC Rule must comply with both that rule and any relevant state breach laws. Given the Web-based business model of many personal health record vendors, this dual compliance may continue to be a substantial source of complication and confusion when breaches occur. Ultimately, it is possible that this can have an unintended negative impact on consumers' responses to breaches. In other words, over-notifying consumers of breaches may result in the "boy who cried wolf" phenomenon.

The FTC Rule creates a rebuttable presumption that unauthorized access to records containing PHI leads to the unauthorized acquisition of that information, but provides the opportunity for regulated entities to demonstrate that the unauthorized access did not in fact lead to improper acquisition (e.g., a laptop is stolen but a forensic analysis indicates that the laptop password was not breached and no information was viewed). Other than this "access/acquisition" distinction, unlike the HHS Rule discussed below, the FTC did not read into the legislation any additional "risk of harm threshold." Instead, in the context of Web-based personal health record vendors, the FTC Rule requires notice in any situation where there has been unauthorized access and the entity cannot demonstrate that no acquisition took place.

The FTC Rule is effective for breaches that take place 30 days[23] after publication in the *Federal Register*. That publication occurred on August 25, 2009, and the rule became effective September 24, 2009; however, sympathetic to industry concerns about the effects of this rule, the FTC has indicated that it will use its enforcement discretion not to seek penalties for compliance failures until a period that is 180 days after the publication of the rule—or five additional months from the compliance date.[24] While announcing this enforcement delay, the FTC also emphasized that it expected full compliance with the requirements from its effective date.[25]

The HHS Rule

The HHS regulation (developed by the HHS Office of Civil Rights, the enforcement agency for the HIPAA Privacy Rule and—in a recent development—the HIPAA Security Rule) was released August 19, 2009, as an "Interim Final Rule." It was published in the August 24, 2009, *Federal Register*.[26] The HHS Rule became effective on September 23, 2009. As noted in Chapter 1, just prior to publication of this book, HHS withdrew the HHS Rule for further consideration. As such, the material discussed herein is subject to change. Until HHS issues a new rule, companies will need to comply with the version of the HHS Rule discussed herein. Because at the time of this writing, the HHS Rule was withdrawn but the new rule was not yet issued, it is important to note that the summary of the HHS Rule discussed herein is subject to change.

While the FTC Rule applies to a relatively limited set of entities, the HHS Rule applies across the health care industry to all HIPAA-covered entities and their business associates. The bulk of the rule deals with the details of notice—relating to timing, the content of the notice, and communication to HHS and the media about breaches.

Under the HITECH Act, breach notification is required only for breaches involving "unsecured" information. In its proposed rule, HHS identified encryption and "destruction" of information as appropriate means of securing information such that the notification "safe harbor" would not require reporting. In the final regulation, HHS reviewed and then rejected various additional means of securing information. Accordingly, to take advantage of this safe harbor, companies must encrypt or destroy information. HHS was quite explicit as to the distinction between appropriate and effective security practices and this safe harbor. For example, HHS directly addressed the concern of some in the health care industry that this rule would mandate encryption. Instead, while encryption clearly is a good practice and is encouraged by HHS in many situations, HHS made clear that there is no overall encryption mandate; instead, companies need to be aware that it is an encryption approach that only permits a company to take advantage of this notification safe harbor. While these other security measures (redaction, limited data sets, etc.) may be effective to reduce any risk of a breach in the first place or the potential harm from a breach, they will not, by themselves, result in application of this safe harbor.

One of the biggest concerns stemming from this provision of the HITECH Act was that companies would be required to provide notice in situations where there was no risk of any harm actually resulting from a disclosure. There was concern both from the covered entity perspective about the costs and potential concerns stemming from disclosures about breaches with no effects, as well as concerns that recipients of these notices would be concerned, confused, or scared about receiving a notice that seemed to describe a "no impact" situation.

Relying on the language of the HITECH Act that concerns notification in situations where a breach "compromised" the privacy or security of health information, and taking a different approach from the FTC, HHS implemented a realistic and responsible "risk of harm" threshold, requiring notice in situations where the incident "poses a significant risk of financial, reputational, or other harm to the individual." The burden of determining that there is no significant risk falls on the covered entity, which otherwise is responsible for notifying the affected individual(s).

The HHS rule also included some interesting discussions about certain activities that might be considered breaches. On the one hand, HHS clarified that only "impermissible" uses and disclosures under HIPAA qualify as breaches. This means, for example, that "incidental disclosures"—certain limited disclosures that may occur despite reasonable precautions (such as one patient overhearing a doctor discuss an issue with another patient)—are permitted under the Privacy Rule and therefore do not qualify as breaches. On the other hand, HHS indicated that a disclosure of "more than" the minimum necessary information might be considered a breach. While covered entities still will apply the "risk of harm" threshold in this context, HHS has focused the industry's attention on some less obvious forms of potential breaches.

State Law

Even though the HITECH Act is set to have an important impact on breaches involving medical information, data breach-notification obligations have been in existence at the state level for several years. The vast majority of states, the District of Columbia, and Puerto Rico have adopted security breach-notification laws that require a person to be notified when certain personal information has been compromised.[27] These numerous laws, while quite similar to one another, do differ in various ways. For the most part, these state laws typically concern types of information that can be used in connection with identity theft (such as Social Security numbers, driver's license numbers, and account numbers). While the majority of states have breach-notification laws for data that can be used to commit financial identity theft, only a small number of states (e.g., California, Arkansas) extend these requirements to health information. California, one of the first states to enact a security breach-notification law, adopted a statute in 2002 that requires that people be notified when their personal information was, or is reasonably believed to have been, acquired by an unauthorized person.[28]

The New York statute, such as the breach-notification laws of many other states, closely follows the California model.[29] Specifically, the New York statute requires that:

[a]ny person or business which conducts business in New York state, and which owns or licenses computerized data which includes private information, shall disclose any breach of the security of the system following discovery or notification of the security of the system to any resident of New York state whose private information was, or is reasonably believed to have been, acquired by a person without valid authorization.[30]

Additionally, the New York statute has a provision that requires any person or business that maintains computerized data that it does not own to notify the owner or licensee of the breach.[31] This is a very important provision, as it enables companies to know of breaches experienced by their vendors and service providers, irrespective of the terms of the underlying vendor contract. The New York breach-notification statute applies to any person or business that conducts business in New York. It does not apply to those entities that collect Social Security numbers (SSNs) of state residents but are not doing business in the state.[32]

Security breach-notification laws were one of the first steps that many states took toward protecting SSNs and preventing identity theft. However, these laws only apply, and help to make people aware, when their SSNs have been or could have been compromised. Security breach-notification laws are not intended to prevent a person's SSN from being compromised in the first place. As such, more recent trends have focused upon measures that aim to help prevent SSNs from ever being compromised.

Other State Laws Imposing Security Requirements

States have begun to play a very important role in regulating data security. Typically, state laws concerning data security cover particular types of data. For example, as will be discussed further below, many states have enacted laws that require entities to provide special protection to SSNs. Other states, including most notably Massachusetts, take matters further and impose specific data security requirements that apply to a wide range of data. The following sections will examine some of these security requirements in further detail.

State Laws Regulating the Use of Social Security Numbers

Over the years, the SSN has become a widely used identifier in both the public and private sectors. Some examples include one's employer for benefit and payroll purposes, banks and other financial institutions that verify identity and check credit using SSNs, courts, tax agencies, and health care insurance companies when a person or their employer enrolls them in a plan. Many state and local governments make the SSNs of certain individuals available in public records.

In the current climate, where data security breaches seem to occur on a daily basis and identity theft is rampant, the widespread use of SSNs and their availability to the public is an issue since these numbers can often be used in connection with various identity theft schemes. To date, despite a number of proposals over the years, the federal government has not passed a comprehensive, uniform law to protect SSNs in the private sector. A number of states, however, have enacted their own laws to protect SSNs in various ways. The different state laws, however, raise problems for some entities, especially companies engaging in any form of interstate commerce, since the laws passed by these states are not uniform and contain varying provisions and requirements.

Many states have enacted laws that limit how SSNs can be maintained and used by both public and private entities. While these laws vary by state, there are some features that many of the laws share, and there are some new trends in state privacy laws.

Quite a few states limit how SSNs can be displayed. For example, Connecticut has implemented a privacy law that restricts the display and use of SSNs.[33] One provision of the Connecticut law provides that no person may "[p]ublicly post or publicly display in any manner an individual's Social Security number,"[34] with "publicly post" and "publicly display" meaning "to intentionally communicate or otherwise make available to the general public."[35] The Connecticut law also has prohibitions against placing an individual's SSN on an identification card, requiring people to send their SSNs over the Internet without proper precautions, and requiring a person to use his or her SSN to access Web sites without other security measures.[36] The law's implications are limited through the definition of "person," however, because it exempts the state, any subdivision of the state, and all state agencies.[37] While this law is helpful in prohibiting the use of SSNs on identification cards and Web sites, the limited applicability to private entities leaves gaps in the protection afforded under the law.

Arizona has also enacted a law to protect SSNs by placing restrictions on their display and use.[38] The Arizona law is an almost identical law to the Connecticut law, except that it adds an additional provision restricting the use of SSNs on items that are mailed to a resident.[39] The Arizona statute, unlike the Connecticut statute, provides some restrictions on the use of SSNs by the state and its subdivisions. Under the statute, SSNs cannot be used by the state or any subdivision of the state on identification cards that they issue.[40] However, the Arizona statute continues to allow agencies of the state and subdivisions of the state to disseminate or use the last four numbers of a person's SSN.[41] The Arizona statute applies to any entity that obtains or maintains the SSNs of Arizona residents.[42]

Minnesota has also enacted a statute that places restrictions on the use and display of SSNs.[43] The Minnesota statute applies to "a person or entity, not including a government entity."[44] Therefore, the Minnesota statute applies only to private entities. The statute contains the provisions of the Connecticut and Arizona statutes pertaining to public posting and use, identification cards, the Internet, and mailings.[45] In addition, the Minnesota statute includes provisions that prohibit "assign[ing] or us[ing] a number as the primary account identifier that is identical to or incorporates an individual's complete Social Security number, except in conjunction with an employee or member retirement or benefit plan or human resource or payroll administration,"[46] and that prohibit selling "Social Security numbers obtained from individuals in the course of business."[47]

Virginia too has a similar statute on the restrictions of SSNs. The Virginia statute prohibits intentionally disclosing a person's SSN, printing an individual's SSN on a card required for obtaining products or services, requiring an SSN to access a Web site unless other security and authorization measures are used, and having an individual's SSN visible in any mailing, whether on the outside or inside of the mailing.[48] Laws such as these, which operate as restrictions on the display and use of SSNs, may help to limit the widespread accessibility of SSNs, thus helping to prevent identity theft.

In addition to the statute covering use and display of SSNs, Connecticut has a public act pertaining to privacy policies applicable to SSNs. Under Public

Act No. 08-167, which became effective on October 1, 2008, any person who collects SSNs in the course of business must create and publicize a privacy policy.[49] The act specifies that the policy must "(1) protect the confidentiality of Social Security numbers, (2) prohibit unlawful disclosure of Social Security numbers, and (3) limit access to Social Security numbers."[50] The act does not apply to any agency or subdivision of the state.[51]

Michigan has a statute that requires a person who obtains one or more SSNs to have a privacy policy that applies to such SSNs.[52] The policy must ensure confidentiality of SSNs, prohibit unlawful disclosure of SSNs, limit who has access to SSNs, describe how to dispose of documents containing SSNs, and establish penalties for violations of the policy.[53] Certain laws, such as the Michigan statute, make an exception for persons or entities that comply with the requirements of the Gramm-Leach-Bliley Act or other federal statutes.[54] Other state laws do not contain such exemptions. Without such an exemption, companies in those states, which are in compliance with applicable federal statutes, may still need to alter their policies and procedures to be in compliance with state laws that place limitations on the use of SSNs.

Several states have adopted laws requiring the state and its subdivisions and agencies to place a privacy policy on their Web sites where personal information, including SSNs, is collected through such sites. One state with such a law is Montana. The Montana statute requires a government operator of a Web site that collects personally identifiable information, which includes SSNs, to ensure that the Web site identifies who operates the Web site, provides contact information for the operator of the Web site, and "generally describes the operator's information practices, including policies to protect the privacy of the user and the steps taken to protect the security of the collected information."[55]

State Laws Imposing Specific Information Security Requirements

Another emerging trend in state privacy laws are statutes that require specific information security requirements and encryption of certain personal data, including SSNs. Nevada is one state that is notable in this regard. First, a Nevada statute that became effective October 1, 2008, requires that "[a] business in this State shall not transfer any personal information of a customer through an electronic transmission other than a facsimile to a person outside of the secure system of the business unless the business uses encryption to ensure the security of electronic transmission."[56] In addition, most recently, as of January 1, 2010, a new measure requires "data collectors" (a broad term that can include businesses and governmental agencies) doing business in the state and that accept payment cards to comply with the payment card industry's security standard known as PCI DSS. Additionally, the new measure also requires data collectors who do not accept payment cards to use encryption when transferring sensitive personal information "outside of the secure system."

Even more notable is Massachusetts. The Massachusetts Office of Consumer Affairs and Business Regulation recently enacted regulations pertaining to identity theft and data security.[57] The regulations have broad coverage since they apply to all entities that "own, license, store, or maintain personal information about a resident of the Commonwealth,"[58] not only those entities that are located or operate in the state. Additionally, the definition of a "person" in the regulations is broad, including "a natural person, corporation, association, partnership, or other legal entity, other than an agency, executive office, department, board, commission, bureau, division, or authority of the Commonwealth, or any of its branches, or any political subdivision thereof."[59] The regulations require that "[e]very person that owns, licenses, stores, or maintains personal information about a resident of the Commonwealth shall develop, implement, maintain, and monitor a comprehensive, written information security program applicable to any records containing such personal information."[60]

The Massachusetts regulations also have provisions governing the encryption of data, including SSNs. The regulations require that all transmitted records and files that contain personal information be encrypted when transmitted wirelessly or over a public network.[61] The regulations also require encryption of all personal information that is "stored on laptops or other portable devices."[62] The Massachusetts statute is one of the broadest encryption laws to have been passed thus far. The new Massachusetts privacy regulations do not contain an exemption for other compliance, such as compliance with HIPAA.

There have been bills for similar laws in other states; for example, lawmakers in the state of Washington have considered a bill that would require the encryption of data.[63] The Washington proposal would add a section that reads "[a]ny person or business that, in the regular course of business and in connection with an access device, collects or stores personal information must comply with payment card industry data security standards established by the PCI security standards council."[64] Also, in Michigan, a Senate bill proposed mandatory encryption of certain data.[65] The Michigan law would add a subsection to Michigan Compiled Laws §445.71,[66] which would state, "[i]f the person collects personal identifying information in the regular course of business and stores that information in a computerized data base, failing or neglecting to store that information in the database in an encrypted form, in conformity with current industry-standard encryption methods and capabilities."[67]

Summary of State Efforts

The Massachusetts regulations are by far the most stringent among state-based efforts to impose information security requirements, but they are not likely to be the last. The Massachusetts data security regulations and bills that have been proposed in other states for similar legislation appear to have been crafted with the primary goal of preventing financial identity theft. However, by impacting data that can also be involved in medical identity theft, such as Social Security numbers and payment information, these laws may also have an important impact on the prevention of medical identity theft. Individuals concerned about the privacy and security of their health information thus have a growing body of laws that may offer protection. Unfortunately, these and other additional protections may be necessary because, as the next section highlights, unauthorized access to medical information remains a major concern.

UNAUTHORIZED ACCESS TO MEDICAL INFORMATION

The discussion of the legal framework applicable to data security may suggest that medical information should be very well protected, and that breaches involving medical information should be few and infrequent. However, this is not the case at all. Rather, medical information continues to be vulnerable in a number of ways. The following sections will examine just how susceptible to unauthorized access and use our medical information can be.

Vulnerability of Medical Information

As we have seen in previous chapters, covered entities and business associates are subject to a very large body of laws and regulations that require them to protect medical information. Furthermore, most entities, especially those involved in the delivery of health care services to consumers, understand that effective data security is a critical part of their business. Accordingly, they have made huge investments in technology to protect data security. And yet, breaches continue to occur.[68] An important factor underlying data insecurities plaguing the health care community can be found in the massive amounts of data and paperwork the health care industry produces in treating an individual, as well as the number of different individuals and entities that may have access to the information. The following sections will examine some of the most significant threats impacting the security of our medical information.

Lost and Stolen Computers and Storage Devices

The loss and theft of laptops and other data-storage devices continue to be major sources of data breaches both inside and outside of the health care sector. There are many examples of cases where an employee of a covered entity left the covered entity's premises with a laptop containing PHI, only to have that laptop lost or stolen, thereby jeopardizing the privacy and security of the PHI stored on that laptop. There have also been many instances where lost and/or stolen laptops or other devices compromised individual patient data. Consider the following examples:

- In 2006, a laptop was stolen from the car of a Kaiser Permanente employee. The laptop was said to contain the names, membership identification numbers, birth-dates, genders, and physician information of 38,000 members of the Kaiser Permanente Plan.[69]

- In February 2009, a researcher's laptop was stolen.[70] The laptop contained the health information of 2,500 subjects who were participating in a study conducted by the National Institutes of Health (NIH).[71]

- In March 2009, personal information from more than 14,000 patients at a North Carolina hospital was compromised when a laptop was stolen from a facility in Canton, Georgia, that was reviewing the information to help the hospital improve care and reduce costs.[72] The laptop was stolen March 9, but the hospital was not alerted to the breach until March 14.[73]

- In August 2009, a laptop was stolen from a hospital employee's car; it contained the private billing information for 33,000 patients of a Florida hospital.[74]

- On November 30, 2009, a laptop containing sensitive patient information was stolen from an employee of the University of California, San Francisco (UCSF) School of Medicine.[75] The laptop contained 4,400 patient records and was not found until January 8, 2010.[76]

Given the high incidence of lost or stolen laptops resulting in major data breaches, many companies, including covered entities, are implementing policies that limit the types of information that can be taken offsite on laptops and other portable devices and/or are mandating encryption for laptops and other portable storage devices upon which certain personal information such as PHI is stored. Both of these methods should have a positive impact on data security.

Data Theft by Medical Workers

Insider criminal actions also present a serious risk to data security. It has been estimated that more than 90 percent of all medical identity theft is attributable to insider theft.[77] The fact that data has become a commodity with a high value may make the theft and resale of such data far too tempting for some employees.

There are a number of notable examples of data theft by medical workers. In 2008, for instance, a former admissions department employee of a New York hospital confessed to stealing the personal information of close to 40,000 patients and then selling that information.[78] Reportedly, an individual seeking personal information for patients born between 1950 and 1970 approached the worker and requested the information. Then, over a period of more than two years, the worker obtained lists of patient names, phone numbers, and Social Security numbers, selling an initial batch of data for $750 and a second batch for $600.[79]

Another example of insider medical identity theft involved a case at the Cleveland Clinic in Weston, Florida, wherein a front-desk office coordinator pleaded guilty to selling information involving more than 1,000 patients.[80] Although the hospital had browser controls to limit the number of records that employees could view, no one noticed the woman was exceeding that limit regularly. The case resulted in $2.8 million in Medicare fraud.[81]

Errors and Mistakes

The privacy and security of medical information is also vulnerable to errors and mistakes by those who are entrusted to protect that information. A very notable case that shows how a simple error can lead to a potentially embarrassing breach occurred in the pre-HIPAA days of 2001. Back then, pharmaceutical giant Eli Lilly became the subject of a Federal Trade Commission (FTC) enforcement action resulting from the security guarantees made in its online privacy policy.[82] Eli Lilly manufactures a number of pharmaceutical products, including the antidepressant Prozac. In marketing Prozac, Lilly operates a Prozac Web site through which it collects various personal data from visitors to the site. From March 2000 to June 2001, Eli Lilly offered a service called Medi-Messenger through its Prozac Web site. The Medi-Messenger service enabled registered users to receive individualized e-mail reminders from Lilly concerning their Prozac medication and other matters.[83] On June 27, 2001, Lilly sent a form e-mail message to the subscribers of the service. The message included in the "To:" entry line the e-mail addresses of every individual subscriber.[84]

The FTC commenced an action against Eli Lilly, alleging that it made false or misleading representations in the privacy policy for the Medi-Messenger service.[85] The privacy policy posted on the Web site at the time the information was collected stated that Eli Lilly employed measures and took steps appropriate under the circumstances to maintain and protect the privacy and confidentiality of personal data obtained from or about consumers through the Prozac site.[86] The FTC alleged that Lilly had not employed such measures or taken such steps. Further, it contended that Lilly failed to provide appropriate training for its employees regarding consumer privacy and information security; failed to provide appropriate oversight and assistance for the employee who sent out the e-mail (an individual who had no prior experience in creating, testing, or implementing the computer program used); and failed to implement appropriate checks and controls on the process, such as reviewing the computer program with experienced personnel and testing the program internally before broadcasting the e-mail.[87]

Eli Lilly eventually settled the matter with the FTC and signed a consent order containing provisions intended to prevent the company from engaging in similar acts and practices in the future.[88] The consent order applies broadly to the collection of personal data from or about consumers in connection with the advertising, marketing, and offering for sale or sale of any pharmaceutical, medical, or other health-related product or service by Eli Lilly.[89] It consists of six parts, but the most significant to the current discussion are parts I and II. Part I of the consent order prohibits misrepresentations regarding the extent to which Lilly maintains and protects the privacy or confidentiality of any personal data collected from or about consumers.[90]

Part II of the consent order requires Eli Lilly to implement a four-stage information-security program designed to protect the confidentiality and security of consumers' personal data and to protect the data against unauthorized access, use, or disclosure.[91] The four stages require Lilly to (i) designate appropriate personnel to coordinate and oversee the program; (ii) identify foreseeable risks to the security, confidentiality, and integrity of personal data, and to address these risks in each relevant area of its operations; (iii) conduct an annual written review by qualified persons that monitors and documents compliance with the program, evaluates its effectiveness, and recommends changes to it; and (iv) adjust the program in light of any findings and recommendations resulting from reviews or ongoing monitoring.[92]

Additionally, there are numerous other examples where errors and mistakes by those entrusted to protect patient information have led to security breaches. In fact, there are multiple examples involving companies failing to secure patient information because of errors and mistakes on many occasions. One such company is insurance giant Kaiser Permanente. In 2005, Kaiser Permanente was fined $200,000 by a California state agency for putting confidential patient information on a Web site in 1999.[93] The California Department of Managed Heath Care concluded that Kaiser created a testing portal Web site containing names, addresses, phone numbers, and even some lab results of nearly 150 patients. The agency claims that Kaiser did not actively work to protect patients until after they had been caught by a former employee and Internet blogger.[94]

Another example involving Kaiser Permanente occurred in 2000 when the insurance giant accidentally sent private e-mail messages that were meant for 858 of its members to 17 unintended members due to a programming glitch.[95] Some of the unintended recipients received hundreds of personal e-mails that included patient addresses, telephone numbers, and answers to sensitive medical questions.[96] Although the problem was realized within 20 minutes and Kaiser Permanente said they contacted the unintended recipients and had the e-mails deleted, it was too late to prevent the breach and highlighted one of the potential problems that can lead to breaches of patient information.[97]

In addition to breaches of patient information occurring from errors and mistakes made by giant companies such as Eli Lilly and Kaiser Permanente, they also occur in smaller organizations. In 2001, 400 pages of documents describing patient visits and diagnoses by therapists of at least 62 children and teenagers were accidentally posted on the University of Montana Web site.[98] In an even smaller setting, but one that still had the potential to harm thousands of individuals, a Nevada woman bought a used computer and found detailed patient information that the previous owner, a drugstore, had failed to delete.[99] These examples show that no matter the size of the company, patient information will always be vulnerable to mistakes and errors.

Snooping

Unauthorized access to medical records also occurs when hospital workers and others access the medical records of celebrities and other well-known individuals. For example, after pop star Britney Spears was hospitalized in 2008 for psychiatric problems, a number of workers at UCLA Medical Center were found to have accessed her records without authorization. In the aftermath of the problem, the hospital fired at least 13 employees and suspended six others for snooping in Spears' confidential medical records.[100]

Other examples include the late country singer Tammy Wynette, the late tennis star Arthur Ashe, and U.S. Congresswoman Nydia Velazquez. A year before her death in 1998, country singer Tammy Wynette had her medical records stolen by a hospital employee who sold them to tabloids for $2,61 0.[101] The employee's position at the hospital entitled him to authorized access to several medical record databases, and he faxed Wynette's records without her consent. The employee was sentenced to six months in prison.[102]

Before his death in 1993, tennis star Arthur Ashe was forced to reveal that he was HIV-positive after a health care worker disclosed his condition without his permission to the newspaper *USA Today*.[103] The newspaper staff contacted Ashe shortly thereafter saying they were going to run the story, forcing Ashe to disclose his condition to the public.[104]

Before being elected to the U.S. House of Representatives, then-New York Congresswoman Nydia Velaquez had her medical records, which included information about an attempted suicide, faxed from a New York hospital to local newspapers and television stations the night before her 1992 primary election.[105] Velazquez won the election and later testified before the Senate Judiciary Committee before the adoption of HIPAA.[106]

Of course, the unauthorized access of medical records is not something that impacts only celebrities and politicians. There have been many instances where an individual who was notable for one reason or another fell victim to the prying eyes of hospital workers who were not authorized to view the person's medical records and did not have any legitimate reason for doing so. For example, in 2006, a seven-year-old child, Nixzmary Brown, tragically died after being tortured and suffering brutal beatings at the hands of her family.[107] The case garnered massive media attention and also the curiosity of hospital workers. Numerous workers at the Woodhull Medical and Mental Health Center accessed her records, allegedly without authorization and/or proper medical purpose. The scope of the unauthorized access was so extensive that 39 employees were suspended without pay for reviewing the child's private medical file.[108] In addition to being subjected to unpaid suspensions from 30 to 60 days, each of the employees found to have accessed the child's medical records without authorization was also required to undergo training in patient privacy rules prior to returning to work.[109]

Snooping can also impact individuals who are not well known in any capacity. If a hospital or other entity does not implement adequate technical controls to prevent it and/or does not train its employees about the dangers of these kinds of behaviors, a curious health worker may access and view medical records of family members, friends, co-workers, and others.

Family Matters

The health care community often ends up being pulled into family conflicts. During divorces and child custody battles, health care providers, pharmacies, and others may find themselves on the receiving end of requests for health information from individuals regarding estranged family members. Health care providers and other HIPAA covered entities have a duty to ensure that the proposed disclosure is legal. For their part, individuals have a responsibility to ensure that their consents are updated to reflect to whom their health information may and may not be disclosed.

Of course, even when all the proper documents are in place, errors still occur. Consider, for example, a California case from 2000.[110] Upon separating from her husband, a woman instructed her pharmacy not to disclose any of her prescription information to him. One day later, the husband contacted the pharmacy for the wife's records, asserting he needed them for tax reasons. The pharmacy complied with the husband's request, turning over all records. Subsequently, the husband disclosed the information to a number of individuals and entities, including the couple's family, friends, and the Department of Motor Vehicles, alleging that his wife was a drug addict and a danger to their children.[111] In the woman's suit against the pharmacy, the pharmacy was found to be at fault because its disclosure of the woman's private information was not in connection with any legal proceeding. As a result of the pharmacy's improper disclosure, a jury awarded the woman $100,000 in damages.[112] Although the woman prevailed in her suit against the pharmacy, her husband was permitted to use the medical records against her because California law permits all relevant information to be submitted as evidence, regardless of how it was obtained or the fact that it may be used for malice or intent to harm, and the husband was initially awarded custody of their children.[113]

Troublingly, there are many other examples of the health care community either being involved in family conflicts or even being the initial cause of them. In a case from 1998, a California-based pharmacy settled with an HIV-positive man after the pharmacist improperly disclosed the man's condition to his ex-wife.[114] The ex-wife was able to use the information to obtain custody of the couple's children.[115] In another case from 1998, a man won a settlement with a Michigan pharmacy after a pharmacy clerk told the man's children that he had AIDS.[116]

Malicious Disclosure of Heath Information

Another highly disturbing recent trend is the unauthorized access to and malicious disclosure of medical information, undertaken for the purpose of maligning, embarrassing, and/or shaming the victim. Unfortunately, there are far too many examples of this shocking behavior. In June 2009, a young mother from Honolulu, Hawaii, was sentenced to a year in prison for illegally accessing another woman's medical records and posting on a MySpace page that the woman was HIV-positive.[117] The state of Hawaii brought charges against the woman under a state statute criminalizing the unauthorized access to a computer, categorizing the conduct of the defendant as a class B felony and sentencing her to a year in jail.[118]

In another shocking case, workers at a medical clinic accessed a patient's medical records and then used them to create a fake MySpace profile that carried the name "Rotten Candy," but included the patient's photo. The profile described "Rotten Candy" as having a sexually transmitted disease, cheating on her husband, and being addicted to plastic surgery.[119]

There is no foolproof way to protect yourself completely against malicious attacks of this nature. Still, you may reduce the likelihood of falling victim to this kind of exposure by selecting covered entities that have comprehensive privacy and security programs, that train employees thoroughly about the necessity for protecting PHI, and that have strong redress mechanisms in place. Still, even with thorough due diligence, there is no guarantee that you will be protected from such outrageous actions. First, you cannot always choose the covered entity that will provide your medical care. While you may choose your own doctor, you may not have the ability to choose your own health insurer, such as in the case of employer-provider health insurance plans. Further, when the need for emergency treatment arises, you may not be able to choose your health care provider. Additionally, these kinds of disclosures can occur even when the covered entity takes your privacy and security very seriously. In each of the cases discussed above, for example, the applicable covered entities appeared to have had implemented comprehensive information-security programs. All it takes, though, is one rogue employee with a vendetta against someone—and access to PHI—to cause a breach that produces lasting harm.

Improper Disposal of Medical Information

Another factor that has a negative impact on heath and medical privacy is the improper disposal of medical information. A health care provider's compliance with HIPAA's privacy and security rules will not be worth a whole lot if, once the provider no longer has a use for the information, it carelessly tosses it in a dumpster, where it can be grabbed by anyone, including identity thieves.

The problems of improper disposal were brought to the public's attention as a result of a major settlement involving the pharmacy CVS.[120] On February 18, 2009, HHS and the Federal Trade Commission (FTC) announced that CVS would pay the government $2.25 million and take corrective action to settle allegations that CVS violated the HIPAA Privacy Rule and the Federal Trade Commission Act.[121]

The regulators' claims that CVS violated HIPAA and the FTC acts arose from allegations that CVS violated the privacy of its prescription customers when it disposed of its customers' information. According to the claims, some CVS employees left labels and other items containing patient information in open trash bins outside stores. News reports claimed that the discarded information included pill bottles, medication instruction sheets, computer order forms, payroll information, job applications, and credit card and insurance information. As a result, regulators asserted that CVS did not have adequate or adequately enforced policies and procedures for disposing of such information, nor did the company sufficiently train its employees to properly handle such material.[122]

After many news reports brought this matter to the public's attention, HHS and the FTC launched a joint investigation into CVS's practices. In addition to HHS's claims regarding HIPAA violations, the FTC alleged that CVS's disposal of data constituted a deceptive business practice under the FTC Act because CVS had claimed to customers that privacy was central to its operations.[123]

The investigation and ensuing settlement are very important for a number of reasons. First, they show that federal regulators are treating the proper disposal of medical information and other sensitive data very seriously, and companies that fail to dispose of sensitive information in a secure manner may face liability. Interestingly, the action also shows that improper disposal of patient health information can create liability under both HIPAA and the FTC acts.

While the proper and safe disposal of PHI has always been an important part of entities' obligations under HIPAA, as a result of the CVS case, HHS posted new guidance on its Web site regarding the proper disposal of patient information.[124] The guidance confirms that the HIPAA Privacy Rule requires covered entities to apply appropriate administrative, technical, and physical safeguards to protect the privacy of PHI. In the guidance, HHS also points out that failing to implement reasonable safeguards to protect PHI in connection with disposal could result in impermissible disclosures of PHI. The guidance instructs covered entities to ensure that each workforce member involved in disposing of PHI, or who supervises those disposing of PHI, must receive training on proper disposal methods.[125]

While the guidance confirms that HIPAA does not require a particular disposal method, it reminds covered entities that they must review their own policies and procedures to make sure they are taking reasonable steps to dispose of PHI. Notwithstanding the foregoing, in the guidance, HHS identifies the following disposal methods as examples of proper disposal methods:[126]

- For PHI in paper records, shredding, burning, pulping, or pulverizing the records so that PHI is rendered essentially unreadable, indecipherable, and otherwise cannot be reconstructed.

- Maintaining labeled prescription bottles and other PHI in opaque bags in a secure area and using a disposal vendor as a business associate to pick up and shred or otherwise destroy the PHI.

- For PHI on electronic media, clearing (using software or hardware products to overwrite media with non-sensitive data), purging (degaussing or exposing the media to a strong magnetic field in order to disrupt the recorded magnetic domains), or destroying the media. Whatever the disposal method selected, a covered entity must ensure that appropriate workforce members receive training and follow the disposal policies and procedures of the covered entity.

MEDICAL ID THEFT

Understanding Medical ID Theft

As the prior section has shown, health information remains vulnerable to a number of serious threats. If data is breached, a number of harms may result, including identity theft. Despite all of the recent emphasis on data security, identity theft continues to be a major problem. A recent FTC report revealed that in 2008, the number of identity theft complaints exceeded 1.2 million, the highest number on record for any particular year since such complaints were tracked.[127] For victims, identity theft is often a life-altering experience that can drain finances, ruin credit, and also take significant emotional, psychological, and physical tolls.

Today, most consumers are aware of the risks of financial identity theft. They also have been educated about the warning signs of such identity theft, as well as some strategies for protecting themselves against this type of crime. There is not, however, a similar level of awareness with respect to the growing threat of medical identity theft. This is most unfortunate because while, like financial identity theft, medical identity theft can lead to financial peril, medical identity theft can also lead to physical harm.

Medical identity theft is said to occur when an individual uses another person's name, sometimes with other parts of that person's identity (such as a Social Security number, insurance card number, or other identification information) without that person's knowledge or consent, in order to obtain medical services or goods.

There are different types of medical ID theft. For example, some acts of medical ID theft result from a single individual seeking medical products or services for which he or she does not have insurance and cannot otherwise afford. Other acts of medical theft may occur in connection with organized crime. Still other acts of theft may be a result of drug addicts seeking prescriptions to narcotics and other controlled substances.[128]

Medical identity theft can result in serious harm. One particular harm that often results is erroneous information being placed into existing medical records. It can also involve the creation of medical records in the victim's name, wherein such medical records reflect the health information of the criminal, not the victim. Often, the erroneous medical records will exist at multiple facilities. As we reviewed earlier in Chapter 2, it can be very time-consuming to change medical records. Further, as we have also reviewed, HIPAA does not provide any right of removal of erroneous medical information. Rather, it only affords individuals the right to amend information in medical records, which is extremely complicated because there is no centralized mechanism for amending medical records. As such, victims will likely need to expend an incredible amount of time corresponding with the applicable medical providers—first to request access to the medical records so that they may be reviewed for accuracy and then to actually request the necessary amendments. Ultimately, the trail of incorrect medical information can impact victims for many years.

Medical identity theft is a crime that is very problematic. After experiencing medical identity theft, a victim will find his or her privacy and security compromised, may have incorrect data in his or her medical records for years to come, and may receive bill after bill for products and services not received. These bills can ultimately impact the individual's credit score and, in turn, his or her ability to get a home, insurance, or even a job.

While individual victims are the most likely to suffer serious consequences from medical identity theft, health care providers and insurers are also victims of medical identity theft. As a result of medical identity theft, health care providers may find themselves providing products and services for which they will never be paid. This results in serious economic loss, some of which is pushed back on all of us through higher premiums and fees. Health care providers victimized by identity theft experience other costs as well. Depending upon the circumstances surrounding the crime, providers may also be subject to heavy penalties and fines, as well as legal expenses and court costs. They may also suffer bad publicity and the loss of goodwill.

Trends in Identity Theft

The risk of medical identity theft may be on the rise. According to a recent report in the *Wall Street Journal*, difficult economic conditions are contributing to an increase in medical identity theft, and the problem is likely to worsen.[129] According to the article, as layoffs leave more and more Americans without health insurance, some individuals are attempting to use someone else's coverage to obtain care.[130] The topics discussed in this article present fundamental questions about health care access—obviously a big issue right now, as potentially wide-ranging health care reform measures are being implemented. At the same time, however, the piece also raises important issues about data security. In a *Wall Street Journal* article, Jilian Mercer reports that the majority of fraud is committed using patient information purchased from health care providers.[131] This fact, along with recent news stories of data theft[132] and data loss[133] in the health care sector, emphasize the need for health care providers and their service providers to reevaluate their current data security policies, procedures, and technical controls to ensure that they are protecting patient data.

Putting It into Context: War Stories

For victims, the consequences of medical identity theft can be profound and long-lasting. While all forms of identity theft can lead to financial ruin and leave individuals feeling victimized and powerless, medical identity theft can be particularly troublesome. The following examples highlight just how troublesome medical ID theft can be.

- **A Pilot Is on the Hook for Surgery He Never Had**
  A pilot from Vail, Colorado, received a collections notice in 2004 for $44,000 in surgery costs from a Denver hospital.[134] He had never visited the hospital in his life. Nevertheless, someone using his name and Social

Security number received extensive treatment and stuck him with the bill. He spent the next two years teetering on the verge of bankruptcy, trying in vain to clear his name.

The massive problems experienced by this pilot had very simple origins, commencing after he placed an ad in an aviation journal. The person taking the order for the ad told the pilot he needed his Social Security number and birth date to verify the check that the pilot had issued for the ad. Unfortunately for the pilot, the person taking the ad was on parole for past crimes and also needed colon surgery. Using the pilot's identity, the ad salesperson got his surgery at a hospital in suburban Denver.[135]

- **A Thief Uses a Marine's Identity to Run Up Medical Charges**

A young marine first learned his life was about to change due to medical identity theft when his mother called to tell him that he was a lead suspect in a South Carolina auto theft case.[136] This young man was not a thief, but he was a victim. He had lost his wallet in South Carolina shortly after completing boot camp. Thereafter, he was posted to California. Meanwhile, in South Carolina, an imposter was living on the marine's identity, using his military ID and driver's license to not only test-drive new cars and then steal them, but also to visit hospitals on several occasions to treat kidney stones and an injured hand, running up nearly $20,000 in medical charges.

The marine found out about the extent of the fraud perpetrated against him when he obtained a credit report following the car theft incident. Reportedly, the victim was not able to get anywhere by pursuing his case with local police. However, a state senator got the U.S. attorney's office in South Carolina involved in his case and, ultimately, the identity thief was arrested. This, however, was not the end of the young marine's difficulties. While he was eventually able to get the hospitals to stop trying to collect on the identity thief's unpaid medical expenses, cleaning up his credit was more complicated and took more time.[137]

- **A Woman Is Billed for the Amputation of a Foot She Still Has**

In early 2004, the 57-year-old owner of a horse farm in Florida received a bill from the local hospital for the amputation of her right foot.[138] The woman, however, was still in possession of both feet. After weeks of fighting with the hospital's billing representatives, she physically went to the hospital to show she was still in possession of her right foot. The hospital eventually dropped the charges, but the woman found out that the mistake was not a billing error. She was the victim of identity theft, and the thief had used her address, Social Security number, and insurance ID number to have the expensive procedure performed.

In addition to having her information stolen, the woman's medical information was now mixed in with the thief's information. When she went to have a hysterectomy performed at the hospital, a nurse looked at her chart and talked to her about the diabetes she did not have.[139] Accordingly, this case illustrates that medical ID theft can result in more than financial harm and can actually lead to medical errors.

- **Newlywed Has Bills From Emergency Room Visits Made around the Country**
  Just before getting married and buying his first home, a 37-year-old manager at an oil and gas company from Houston, Texas, requested a copy of his credit report in order to apply for a mortgage. Upon receiving the report, he found out that he had thousands of dollars in collection notices listed under his name for emergency rooms trips from across the country. Having never before actually gone to the emergency room, he discovered he too was the victim of medical identity theft.[140]
  Included in the list of charges made using the man's identity was a $19,000 bill for an ambulance service in a part of the country he had never heard of and emergency rooms bills from the likes of Kansas. Six years after discovering he was a victim of medical identity, the Houston man was still dealing with the fallout.[141]

New Legal Weapons against ID Theft

Given the incidence and consequences of identity theft, it is not surprising that legislators, consumer protection agencies, and advocates continue to seek new ways to prevent identity theft and mitigate the effects when it does occur. The enactment of the "red flag rules" (the Rules)[142] is one important initiative designed to help control the growth of identity theft. The Rules require financial institutions and creditors to assist the government in detecting, preventing, and mitigating red flags of identity theft. The FTC defines a red flag as a "pattern, practice, or specific activity that indicates the possible existence of identity theft."[143] For example, if a physician covered by the Rules requires patients to produce copies of insurance cards and a patient produced a card that appeared fake, forged, or altered, that may be a red flag.

The Rules are of relevance to the present discussion because they define "creditor" broadly[144] in a manner that would cover many physicians. The American Medical Association and other groups, however, have been endeavoring to convince the FTC that it is incorrect to include physicians under the scope of the Rules. While, as noted above, the implementation of the Rules has been delayed several times, physicians have not yet been excluded from the obligation to comply with the Rules. For those who are subject to them, a failure to comply may result in both civil monetary penalties and less tangible losses, such as negative publicity and the loss of goodwill.

While the Rules will apply to many physicians, they will not impact all. The duty to comply will hinge on whether a physician's activities fall within the law's definition of two key terms: "creditor" and "covered account."[145] Physicians will be subject to the Rules if they satisfy a two-part test. First, the provider must be a creditor. Under the broad definition of creditor, a physician who renders medical services to a patient without taking full payment at the time of service but rather defers payment by billing the patient will be a creditor. The same holds true for a physician who renders medical services to a patient and accepts the patient's co-pay.[146]

Under the second part of the test to be subject to the Rules, a physician must offer or maintain covered accounts for patients. According to the Rules, a covered account is one in which a creditor offers or maintains for personal, family, or household purposes, and that involves multiple payments or transactions, and any other account that the creditor offers or maintains for which there is a reasonably foreseeable risk to patients of identity theft.[147] A physician who is a creditor must have a continuing relationship with the patient before the patient's account is considered a covered account.

Pursuant to the Rules, physicians who are creditors offering or maintaining covered accounts are required to develop, implement, and maintain a written identity theft prevention program designed to detect, prevent, and mitigate identity theft. At a minimum, the Rules require that the program provide policies and procedures to (i) identify relevant red flags and incorporate them into the program; (ii) detect red flags in patient accounts; (iii) respond appropriately to any red flags detected in patient accounts; and (iv) ensure the program is updated periodically to reflect changes in risks to patients and the safety and soundness of the physician from identity theft, each as discussed further below.[148]

Identify red flags: A physician who is subject to the Rules must implement a program to identify patterns, practices, or specific activities that indicate the possible risks of identity theft. These items are known as "red flags." There is no "one-size-fits-all" approach to identifying red flags. Covered physicians, as well as all others who are covered by the Rules, must identify those red flags that are relevant to their particular practice or business. In doing so, the physician must consider certain factors, such as (i) which of its accounts are subject to the risk of identity theft; (ii) the methods it provides to open its accounts; (iii) the methods it provides to access its accounts; (iv) its size, location, and patient base; and (v) its previous experiences with identity theft.

Detect red flags: Physicians covered by the Rules must also establish and implement policies and procedures to detect those red flags in their day-to-day operations. Red flags may be identified in a number of different areas of practice. For example, a physician may identify a red flag when verifying a patient's identity, monitoring certain transactions, and/or processing changes of address.

Respond to red flags: The compliance program must be commensurate with the degree of risk posed and address the risk of identity theft to the individual patient and the financial institution or physician. The regulation provides an illustrative list of appropriate measures that may be used to respond to red flags. Some examples are:

1. Monitoring an account for evidence of identity theft;
2. Contacting the applicable patient;
3. Changing any passwords, security codes, or other security devices that permit access to a patient's account;
4. Reopening an account with a new account number;
5. Not opening a new account;
6. Closing an existing account;
7. Notifying law enforcement;
8. Implementing any requirements regarding limitations on credit extensions;
9. Implementing any requirements for furnishing of information to consumer reporting agencies; and
10. Determining that no response is warranted under the circumstances.

Updating the program: Of course, it will not be sufficient to simply have a written policy in place. The policy will only be as effective as the physician's efforts to ensure that the policy is complied with. The physician should periodically update the program, considering his or her own experiences with identity theft, changes in the methods of identity theft, changes in methods to detect, prevent, and mitigate identity theft, changes in accounts offered and maintained, and changes in business arrangements. In addition, as is essential with all effective privacy and data security programs, physicians implementing a program to comply with the Rules must train staff to implement the program and exercise appropriate and effective oversight of it.

Time will tell how effective the Rules will be in preventing identity theft. However, it is interesting to note that there is this new tool in the arsenal against identity theft. From the patient's perspective, you may expect that as physicians implement programs to comply with the Rules, you may be asked to provide various forms of identification to your treating physician. If this matter is of concern to you, you should feel free to ask your doctor what they are doing to comply. There also remains a question of whether the red flags rules will continue to apply to medical professionals. On May 21, 2010, the American Medical Association, the American Osteopathic Association, and the Medical Society of the District of Columbia filed a lawsuit against the FTC in U.S. District Court for the District of Columbia in an attempt to prevent the FTC from extending identity theft regulations to physicians.[149] The medical societies argue that the Rules exceed the FTC's powers delegated to it by Congress, and its application to physicians is "arbitrary, capricious, and contrary to the law."[150]

"This unjustified federal regulation of medicine treats physician practices like banks, credit card companies, and mortgage lenders," said AMA President-elect Cecil B. Wilson, MD. "The extensive bureaucratic burden of complying with the red flags rule outweighs any benefit to the public."[151]

Additionally, the suit claims that physicians are already ethically and legally responsible for ensuring the confidentiality and security of patients' medical information, and as such, the Rules are an additional unnecessary regulation.[152]

This lawsuit comes after more than two years of communications between the physicians' representatives and the FTC regarding the unintended consequences of the regulations, and was brought only after the FTC responded on March 25, 2010, stating that the Rules would apply to physicians.[153]

Although the suit came before the Rules were to apply, it does not delay the Rules' effect date, and physicians are required to comply until a decision is granted in their favor, if that ends up being the ultimate outcome.[154]

In addition to the lawsuit, Congress has gotten involved. On October 20, 2009, the House of Representatives overwhelmingly passed H.R. 3763, which exempts "any health care practice, accounting practice, or legal practice with 20 or fewer employees from the meaning of creditor subject to red flag guidelines regarding identity theft." The measure went to the Senate on October 21, 2009, and was referred to the Senate Banking Committee. The Senate, however, has not yet acted on the bill.[155] Meanwhile, the FTC has delayed the implementation of the Rules yet again. At the time of this writing, the Rules were scheduled to enter into force on December 31, 2010.

Protecting Yourself against Medical ID Theft

Although there are important legislative tools that aim to prevent identity theft, we as consumers cannot sit back and expect legislators to protect us completely, nor can we expect for our providers to be able to detect all potential fraudsters and protect us against identity theft. Lawmakers and health care providers have an important role to play in our protection, but we do as well. While not all instances of medical identity theft can be prevented, there are certain steps you can take to protect yourself. The list below identifies examples of risk-management strategies that you might consider implementing to better protect yourself from identity theft. In addition, Exhibit A contains a checklist for responding to identity theft.

- Keep track of all of your medical providers and obtain copies of your medical records so that you can review them for accuracy and so that, if they are tampered with in the future, you will have a point of reference as to what they contained as of a certain date.

- Request an accounting of disclosures from your providers on a regular basis so that you may see who has accessed your medical records.

- Store health insurance and prescription benefit cards in a safe location. Treat these cards as you would treat your credit or debit cards.

- On an annual basis, request a complete list of annual payments that your insurance company has made for your care. This may help you to uncover cases where an identity thief has changed your billing address in order to receive payments at a different address. Sometimes, medical identity thieves will obtain care using a different address from the victim's actual address so that the victim will not become aware of the charges being made.

- Review carefully all correspondence from your insurer. Examine all statements to ensure that they do not contain any treatments and/or services that you did not receive.

- If you note errors or suspect you have been the victim of identity theft, immediately contact the physician and request that your file be amended.

- If you receive Medicaid or Medicare and suspect that you have been a victim of medical identity theft, promptly contact your regional office of the Centers for Medicare & Medicaid Services.

- Monitor your credit report, looking for reports of debts that you have not incurred that may be related to someone else's medical expenses.

CONCLUSION

The security of data will continue to grow in importance as the health care industry moves toward greater implementation of electronic health records. Congress has already proposed numerous bills to facilitate and regulate that transition. At the same time, however, advances in information technology will likely make it easier to implement enhanced technical security measures such as audit trails and access controls in the future.

Personal health records may be an option for individuals who wish to take greater control over their own medical information. However, personal health records are not without pitfalls and areas of concern. The next chapter will examine the fundamentals of personal health records. While examining their utility for patients seeking more control over their own medical information, this chapter will also explore key legal and practical considerations that consumers should take into account when contemplating the creation, maintenance, and use of PHRs.

4

Taking It into Your Own Hands: Personal Health Records

INTRODUCTION

It's a typical morning at home. Everyone is rushing about to get to where they need to be on time. As the mom, inevitably, all of the loose ends fall to you. As you are seeing your youngest child off to the school bus, your eldest daughter is yelling about her missing vaccination records. She is nearly in tears now, whining that she will not be allowed to play soccer with her team unless she can produce the records of her most recent vaccination. Meanwhile, your husband is yelling downstairs to you, asking if you have seen his report from his recent MRI. He has an appointment with the chiropractor during his lunch break, and he says it will be useless if he cannot bring in his MRI report. You cringe as you hear him banging around upstairs, knowing that he is tearing apart the recently cleaned home office in search of his report. Meanwhile, you remember that you have agreed to take your father to his doctor's appointment after work and note that you will need to bring in a full list of his medications.

Instead of feeling overwhelmed in the midst of this mini-crisis, you make a second cup of coffee for yourself, open your laptop, and log on to the personal health record you have created for your family. Within minutes, you pull up Stephanie's vaccination report, print a copy, and then hurry her out the door and off to school. Next up, you e-mail your husband his MRI report, while at the same time requesting that the system send him a text message letting him know the record is in his e-mail. This saves you from yelling up to him or having to run upstairs to tell him. Finally, you log into your parents' personal health record, compile a full list of your father's prescriptions, and then e-mail it to his doctor. With that done, you are now ready for the challenges of the workday ahead, and you head out to the office.

Does this all sound too good to be true? Well, it's not. Thanks to personal health records, this very scenario can play out at your breakfast table tomorrow morning. But there are some areas of concern about this brave new world of personal health records (PHRs). Providers of electronic PHRs are generally not subject to the same privacy and security obligations as a health care provider, and some may not offer sufficient technical security. What's more, certain information stored in a PHR may be accessible by third parties, including the PHR provider's business partners and service providers—and in some cases, even government agencies.

Fortunately, there are ways to minimize risk if you choose to create a personal health record. With this in mind, this chapter aims to guide you on how you might make positive use of PHRs, while reducing the likelihood of unanticipated exposure.

Although PHRs have been getting a fair amount of public attention in recent months, the concept is far from new. Personal health records have existed for as long as people have been maintaining files of lab reports and other medical records. But today's Web-based and electronic PHR options are providing individuals with greater control over their medical information. By assembling and maintaining personal health records, people can reduce the risks of medical errors, control costs, and play a significant role in managing their and their family's health care.

However, while Web-based and electronic PHRs offer consumers several benefits, it is important to note that they also raise issues of security and privacy. After examining personal health records and exploring how they are regulated, this chapter will discuss techniques for maximizing the benefits and minimizing the risks of personal health records.

UNDERSTANDING PERSONAL HEALTH RECORDS

What Is a Personal Health Record?

A personal health record refers to a health or medical record that is initiated and maintained by an individual, as opposed to a third party, such as a medical provider or insurer. PHRs can apply to both paper-based and electronic records; however, in the current era, the term is usually used to refer to an electronic, Web-based application.

PHRs can be used to store a wide range of health and medical information. Some may focus on specific issues, such as vaccination records and/or medications, while many provide means for organizing a variety of data. Those that are more comprehensive typically provide a means for tracking medications (including dosage information and adverse reactions), allergies, illnesses, surgeries and hospitalization records, test results, vaccinations, and family history information. Many electronic PHRs provide additional services that go beyond merely compiling data. For example, some allow individuals to communicate with their health care providers, check interactions among certain drugs and other substances, and conduct research on medical conditions.

PHRs are available through a number of different channels. Some PHRs are marketed directly to consumers. In this scenario, the provider may or may not charge usage or subscription fees. Those that are free often generate fees through other sources, like advertising or promotions. Other PHRs may be offered by hospitals or health plans. Technology powerhouses, including Google Health, Microsoft HealthVault, WebMD, and Revolution Health, run some of the more popular PHRs.

Additionally, PHRs can be established and maintained in a number of different formats, including a paper-based PHR, which may include printouts of laboratory tests, procedures, conditions, and other health-related information, usually maintained in one's home. A paper-based PHR, however, has a number of limitations. It is usually only accessible in a single location and is vulnerable to theft, loss, and natural disasters like floods and fires.

Another option is a PC-based PHR, with health and medical information stored locally on an individual's personal computer. A PC-based PHR can be as simple as a collection of documents in a word-processing program. However, more sophisticated PC-based PHRs may employ data encryption. PC-based PHRs, however, are also subject to some of the same limitations as the paper-based system—loss, physical corruption, and damage.

As such, most contemporary PHRs are Internet-based and allow individuals to access and edit their medical records via a Web site. The data is stored remotely on a single server controlled by the PHR vendor and/or its service provider. Internet-based PHRs are typically more robust and offer greater functionality than PC-based PHRs.

Depending on the PHR vendor and the commitments that it makes to data security, integrity, and business continuity, data stored with an Internet-based PHR may be less vulnerable to physical loss and damage than those stored via paper or on a local computer. However, they are far from immune, particularly if the PHR vendor uses a single server or lacks an adequate backup plan.

Still, one of the main advantages of Internet-based PHRs is that they allow for greater interactivity. When PHRs are stored on the Web, individuals are better able to share them with family members, physicians, and others who are involved in their health and care. Of course, this high level of interactivity may also result in greater vulnerability to unauthorized access. For these reasons, it is critical for individuals to have a full understanding of a vendor's privacy and security commitments and capabilities.

As personal technology evolves at a rapid pace, so do electronic records; with the latest form of PHRs, health information can even be stored on your smartphone or iPhone. There are many iPhone applications that allow you to create and manage a PHR, and a number of Internet-based PHRs offer smartphone-based versions of their services.

What Are the Advantages of PHRs?

The advantages of PHRs go beyond the personal convenience of being able to quickly and easily access medical records, which is of course a major advantage in itself. Having a PHR and sharing information from it with a health care provider allows the patient and provider to work together cooperatively. It can also help to reduce or eliminate duplicate procedures or tests; a physician may be able to access the results of a test recently ordered by another physician instead of ordering the test to be conducted again. This, in turn, can save time and reduce unnecessary medical expenditures.

PHRs also give medical consumers a new level of control over their care and can foster better decision making. For instance, when records regarding cholesterol levels and blood pressure remain locked away in the doctor's office, the patient is removed from tracking and understanding her health. However, when a patient maintains her own records, she is able to assume a more active role in monitoring her health and behaviors.

How Are PHRs Regulated?

Overview

As discussed earlier, the Health and Insurance Portability and Accountability Act (HIPAA) applies only to particular entities, namely covered entities and their business associates. There is no federal privacy law that protects health information in other contexts and/or processes by other entities. Most entities that are involved in collecting, storing, using, or processing PHRs are not covered by HIPAA. Whether HIPAA applies to a PHR vendor depends on whether that vendor is a covered entity itself or a business associate to a covered entity. As mentioned earlier, some PHRs are offered by health providers, such as hospitals or health plans, that are covered entities and are therefore bound by the HIPAA Privacy Rule[1] and the HIPAA Security Rule.[2]

While some PHRs are offered by covered entities, many PHRs are sponsored by third parties from outside the health care system and are not subject to HIPAA. Nonetheless, some of these PHRs may claim to be HIPAA compliant. You should investigate any such claim very carefully before relying on it, as an entity cannot be HIPAA compliant if it is not subject to HIPAA and its audit and enforcement powers. A PHR vendor that claims HIPAA compliance may mean it has implemented policies and procedures that are consistent with HIPAA's Privacy and Security Rule. However, claims of HIPAA compliance should not be construed as guarantees of privacy and security.

Microsoft takes an interesting and progressive point of view on the regulation of its HealthVault service. Initially, the company claimed that HealthVault was not a covered entity or business associate, as the service provided tools to help individuals manage copies of their own health information.[3] But this position was altered somewhat in June of 2009, when Microsoft made this announcement:

. . . ambiguity and uncertainty surrounding new health privacy provisions in the American Recovery and Reinvestment Act of 2009 have raised new questions about whether HIPAA applies to services offered by covered entities that connect to consumer-driven online health platforms like HealthVault. We do not want this ambiguity and uncertainty to stall progress toward a dynamic, trusted patient-centric health care system. Microsoft is also committed to complying with applicable laws. That is why we offer HealthVault solution providers that are HIPAA covered entities the opportunity to sign our HealthVault business associate agreement.[4]

In the announcement, Microsoft is not "admitting" that it is a business associate and is, in fact, expressly denying that it is a covered entity.[5] But the company wanted to step forward on privacy issues in an apparent effort to move beyond protracted negotiations about the classification of its services. Blogging on this point, a Microsoft representative commented:

So we decided to take a new look at the legislation. And when we did that, we realized that it really didn't matter how we are technically defined. As we have said from day one, we operate the HealthVault systems far beyond the baseline privacy and security measures required by HIPAA anyways. And further, we can sign business associate agreements with covered entities that want to interact with HealthVault, without in any way restricting our ability to put consumers in control of their information. To be clear—we can and will, without modification or compromise, continue to stand behind our privacy statement and service agreement.[6]

Enforcement of Privacy Policies of PHR Vendors

PHR providers are required to comply with their stated privacy policies. Failing to comply with one's stated privacy can result in legal actions by the Federal Trade Commission (FTC) and state authorities. It can also raise the possibility of private lawsuits, including class actions.

There have been a number of cases outside of the world of PHRs that clearly demonstrate that companies will be bound by the terms of their stated policies. Such cases are of particular importance when one considers the kinds of demands for information that governmental authorities have been making on private entities, including requiring such companies to disclose customer data to the government, even when doing so would cause the companies to be in violation of their own policies.

The FTC's power as an agency that enforces privacy promises emerged back in 2000 and has been growing ever since. In July 2000, the FTC commenced an enforcement action against bankrupt online toy store Toysmart .com, LLC, and Toysmart.com, Inc. (Toysmart).[7] The FTC was alerted when, in conjunction with its dissolution, Toysmart attempted to sell personal data collected via the Internet, even though the privacy policy posted at the time the personal data were collected assured customers that the information collected from them would never be shared with third parties. On May 22, 2000, Toysmart announced that it was closing its operations and selling its assets. Despite the assurances in Toysmart's privacy policy, the company offered personal data collected via its Web site as part of the assets it was selling.[8]

As a result of Toysmart's actions, the FTC initiated an enforcement action against the company, charging that it had violated Section 5 of the FTC Act by misrepresenting to customers that personal data would never be shared with third parties and then disclosing, selling, and offering for sale that personal data in violation of the company's stated privacy policy.[9]

This action eventually ended in a settlement pursuant to which Toysmart was prohibited from selling its customer list as a stand-alone asset.[10] The settlement permitted Toysmart to sell such customer lists containing personal data only (1) as part of a package that included the entire Web site, (2) to an entity that was in a related market, and (3) to an entity that expressly agreed to be Toysmart's successor-in-interest as to the personal data. Under the terms of the settlement, the buyer of Toysmart's assets would have to agree to abide by Toysmart's privacy policy and to obtain the affirmative consent (opt-in) of the data subjects prior to using their personal data in any manner that was inconsistent with Toysmart's original privacy policy.[11]

Toysmart's difficulties with the FTC illustrate the hazards of posting a privacy policy that is not completely accurate. For Toysmart, as well as many other companies of a similar nature, personal data is a major asset. By drafting a privacy policy in a very restrictive manner, Toysmart effectively limited its business plan and was not able to use one of its primary assets as it had intended. When the company attempted to transfer the personal data it had collected in contravention of its privacy policy, the FTC had prevented it from doing so.

Since this early case in 2000, there have been a number of cases that showed that regulators will take action against companies that fail to act in accordance with their stated policies.

More recently, the FTC has begun to focus on those companies that have failed to honor their commitments to data security or, irrespective of what they have promised, have failed to protect data security. For example, the FTC brought enforcement actions against software giant Microsoft[12] and accessory clothing manufacturer Guess for making false assurances regarding the level of security they provided to individuals' personal data.[13] In this most recent case, the FTC alleged that clothing manufacturer Guess failed to use reasonable or appropriate measures to protect consumers' personal data, and thereby exposed consumers' information to commonly known attacks by hackers, all in contravention with Guess's assurances that the data collected through its Web site would be protected.[14]

Guess has sold clothing and accessories through its Web site at http://www.guess.com since 1998. The FTC alleged that since October 2000, the company's Web site had been vulnerable to a number of commonly known Web-based application attacks. According to the FTC, despite these attacks, Guess's online statements assured consumers that their information would be protected.[15] Specifically, according to the FTC, at the time the Guess Web site was attacked, it contained the following statements: "This site has security measures in place to protect the loss, misuse and alteration of information under our control" and "All of your personal information, including your credit card information and sign-in password, are stored in an unreadable, encrypted format at all times."[16] The FTC alleged that, despite these assurances, Guess did not store consumers' information in an unreadable, encrypted format at all times and, in fact, the security measures implemented by Guess failed to protect against structured query language (SQL) and other commonly known attacks.[17]

The eventual settlement agreement between Guess and the FTC prohibited Guess from misrepresenting the degree to which it protects the security of personal information collected from consumers. It also required Guess to establish and maintain a comprehensive data security program. Furthermore, Guess is also required to have its security program certified annually by an independent security professional.[18]

The FTC also entered into a consent agreement with PETCO Animal Supplies, Inc. after the FTC alleged that PETCO had engaged in deceptive trade practices by including various statements in its online privacy policy,[19] including:

At PETCO.com, protecting your information is our number one priority, and your personal information is strictly shielded from unauthorized access. Entering your credit card number via our secure server is completely safe. The server encrypts all of your information; no one except you can access it.[20]

The FTC alleged that these statements were a deceptive trade practice because PETCO was unable to completely protect the data it received from its computer servers.[21] The FTC settlement prohibited PETCO from misrepresenting the extent to which it maintains and protects sensitive consumer information. It also required PETCO to establish and maintain a comprehensive information-security program designed to protect the security, confidentiality, and integrity of personal information collected from or about consumers.[22] It required that

PETCO arrange biennial audits of its security program by an independent third party certifying that Petco's security program is sufficiently effective to provide reasonable assurance that the security, confidentiality, and integrity of consumers' personal information has been protected. The settlement also contained recordkeeping provisions to allow the FTC to monitor compliance."[23]

In 2004, the FTC targeted and entered into a consent agreement with Gateway Learning Corporation.[24] The FTC alleged that Gateway had engaged in unfair and deceptive trade practices by sharing customer information collected after explicitly promising on its Web site not to do so.[25] Initially, the Gateway privacy policy stated, "We do not sell, rent, or loan any personally identifiable information regarding our consumers with any third party unless we receive the customer's explicit consent."[26] Gateway then decided to sell customer information collected on its Web site and altered its privacy policy to state that "from time to time" Gateway would provide consumers' personal information to "reputable companies" whose products or services consumers might find of interest.[27]

The FTC charged that (1) Gateway's claims that it would not sell, rent, or loan to third parties consumers' personal information unless it received the consumers' consent, and that it would never share information about children, were false; (2) Gateway's retroactive application of a materially changed privacy policy to information it had previously collected from consumers was an unfair practice; and (3) Gateway's failure to notify consumers of the changes to its privacy policy and practices, as promised in the original policy, was a deceptive practice.[28] The settlement barred misrepresentations about how Gateway will use data it collects from consumers. It prohibited Gateway from sharing any personal information collected from consumers on its Web site under the earlier privacy policy unless it first obtains express affirmative, or "opt-in," consent from consumers, and prohibited it from applying future material changes to its privacy policy retroactively without consumers' consent. Further, the settlement also required Gateway to give up the $4,608 it earned from renting consumers' information.[29]

In April 2005, the FTC settled charges against BJ's Wholesale Club.[30] According to the complaint, the FTC alleged that BJ's use of its computer network to obtain bank authorization for credit and debit card purchases and to track inventory was not reasonably secure to protect customer information. For credit and debit card purchases at its stores, BJ's collects information, such as name, card number, and expiration date, from the magnetic stripe on the back of the cards. The information is sent from the computer network in the store to BJ's central data center computer network, and from there through outside computer networks to the bank that issued the card. The FTC charged that BJ's engaged in a number of practices that, taken together, did not provide reasonable security for sensitive customer information.[31]

These practices included (1) BJ's failure to encrypt consumer information when it was transmitted or stored on computers in its stores; (2) BJ's creation of unnecessary risks to the information by storing it for up to 30 days; and (3) storing the information in files that could be accessed using commonly known default user IDs and passwords.[32] As a result of the settlement, BJ's was required to establish and maintain a comprehensive information-security program that includes administrative, technical, and physical safeguards[33] BJ's was also required to obtain an audit from a qualified, independent, third-party professional verifying that its security program meets the standards of the order and to comply with standard bookkeeping and recordkeeping provisions.[34]

FTC Breach-Notification Rule

While some PHR vendors may not have to comply with HIPAA, they do have to comply with the FTC's Health Breach Notification Rule (the FTC Breach Rule).[35] Meanwhile, the FTC Breach Rule does not apply to HIPAA covered entities or their business associates, which must comply with the breach-notification rule issued by HHS.[36] Entities subject to the FTC Breach Rule who experience a "breach" of unsecured identifiable health information are to notify (1) the individuals whose information was breached, and (2) the FTC, or in the case of third-party service providers providing services to PHR vendors or related entities, the service provider is to notify the applicable PHR vendor or related entity, which must then notify the FTC.[37]

Like the HHS Rule, the FTC Rule imposes specific requirements for breach notices, specifically:

Timing of notification: The FTC breach rule requires that notice be made to impacted individuals "without reasonable delay" and in no case more than 60 calendar days after the discovery of the breach. If the breach impacts more than 500 individuals, notice must be made to the FTC within 10 business days after the discovery of the breach. If it affects more than 500 residents of a particular state or jurisdiction, prominent media outlets in that state or jurisdiction must also be alerted. A log of breaches impacting fewer than 500 people must be maintained and submitted to the FTC annually no later than 60 days following the end of the calendar year.[38]

Method of notification: Companies must send a notice to an individual's last known address via first-class mail or by e-mail if the individual has agreed in advance to be contacted electronically. If the contact information for 10 or more individuals is found to be outdated or insufficient, the entity must provide substitute notice in one of the following forms:

• Conspicuous posting on the home page of its Web site for at least 90 days; or

• In major print or broadcast media in the areas where the impacted individuals likely reside. In this case, the notice must include a toll-free number that people can call to learn whether they have been affected by the breach. The phone number must remain active for at least 90 days.[39]

Content of notice: Notices sent to individual consumers must be in "plain language" and include:

- A brief description of what happened, including the date of the breach and the date the breach was discovered (if known);
- A description of the types of unsecured identifiable health information involved in the breach;
- Steps individuals should take to protect themselves from potential harm that may result from the breach;
- A brief description of what the entity is doing to investigate the breach, mitigate harm, and protect against future breaches; and
- Contact procedures for individuals to ask questions or obtain additional information.[40]

State Requirements

In addition to the notification requirements of the Health Information Technology for Economic and Clinical Health Act (HITECH),[41] the majority of states have enacted their own breach-notification laws. However, only a small number of those laws apply to health information. When the notification requirements of the FTC Breach Rule conflict with the notification requirements of a particular state, the FTC Breach Rule takes precedence under the preemption clause contained in the HITECH Act. However, entities subject to state laws imposing additional or more stringent notification requirements must comply with those requirements as well.

CONCERNS ABOUT PHRS

Privacy Concerns

PHRs raise a number of potential privacy and security concerns, such as the vendor's ability to access and use the information. For example, some companies may "mine" the PHRs they host and sell data to advertisers or other third parties. For some, this will not be problematic and may be viewed as an acceptable trade-off for the free use of the vendor's system. However, others may view any analysis and sale of their information—even that which is strictly anonymous—as an unacceptable privacy violation.

But some PHR vendors go beyond offering anonymous health information and sell your contact information to marketers who are focused on issues surrounding conditions you have. For example, if you have hypertension, you may be contacted about new treatments, products, and services that are used to lower blood pressure. Some who are troubled by this may view the receipt of such unsolicited marketing as a minor annoyance and a trade-off for the use of the service. Others may even view targeted advertisements as valuable, especially if those ads offer access to goods and services that are helpful with respect to the treatment and management of their illness. However, some may have mistakenly assumed their information wouldn't be shared with third parties and may view this activity as a violation of their privacy.

Individuals have different expectations and tolerance levels for the use of their medical information by third parties. Likewise, PHRs have a wide range of policies and procedures with respect to the collection, use, and disclosure of data that is stored with them. Medical consumers contemplating the possible use of a PHR must review the policies of the PHR vendor very carefully before signing up for the service and certainly prior to sharing any medical information. This will be discussed further in "Choosing a PHR Vendor."

Additionally, you should note that if a company hosting a PHR is served a subpoena, it may share your information regardless of the privacy policies put in place regarding typical third parties. If you are interested in storing your information with a PHR vendor, you should review and understand their policies for complying with subpoenas and other official demands for information.

Security Concerns

A predominant concern surrounding PHRs is security. When you store your medical information with a third party, you are entrusting some of your most private and personal information to that provider. How can you be sure that your information will be protected from hackers and electronic intrusions? Since PHR vendors that are not covered entities or business associates don't have to comply with the HIPAA Security Rule, the obligation falls on you to investigate and understand what the vendor will and will not do to protect sensitive information.

Without proper security, medical information can fall into the hands of a variety of unauthorized recipients, including identity thieves and other criminals. Individuals involved in special situations may have specific concerns about the security of their medical records. For example, an individual involved in a personal-injury lawsuit might be particularly concerned about the security of his or her medical records. Similarly, a person suffering from an addiction or a disease that is the subject of social stigma may be interested in ensuring the security of his or her medical information.

Consider, for instance, if you had an ailment or were seeking certain treatments that you did not wish to be disclosed to an insurer. You might pay for the treatments in cash and would not seek reimbursement for your costs from your insurer. However, seeking to monitor how your body responds to the treatments, you upload your data to a PHR. You will want to be sure that the vendor of that PHR is capable of protecting the security of your information. The next section of this chapter, "Choosing a PHR Vendor," will explore key considerations for selecting a provider for your PHR. At the end of the day, it is your responsibility to read and understand the vendor's policies and agreements before you entrust the provider with your business—and your most private information.

Terminated and Inactive Accounts

There are serious concerns over the issue of inactive accounts and the termination of vendor operations. While there is a lot of promise for the future of the sector, at present the PHR market is still quite immature and is in a state of rapid evolution. It is likely that some of today's PHR vendors will not survive or will be bought out by larger enterprises. At the same time, given the novelty and continued development of the industry, there are very real concerns about consumer loyalty to particular PHR vendors. Consumers interested in maintaining their own PHRs may jump around, switching vendors when a new vendor emerges or an existing one offers new functionality, a more user-friendly interface, or valuable sign-up promotions. Others may find that maintaining their own PHR was more work than they had anticipated and drop off completely.

In each of these scenarios, the end result may be that a vendor (which may or may not be the original vendor you had signed up with) may be in possession of inactive accounts replete with medical information. Another potential issue is the possible wholesale deletion of PHRs by a company that goes out of business or is bought by another entity.

There are some ways to reduce the risks of these kinds of occurrences. First, you might consider choosing an established provider, which may increase the likelihood that the provider will remain in business. You should also research the provider's policies and make sure you understand what they will do with your data in the event that you terminate or cease to use your account.[42] The provider's policies may also clarify what the provider will and will not do in the event of a merger, acquisition, or similar transaction. You may also wish to maintain digital and/or paper backups of your information so that, in the worst-case scenario, you will not need to recreate your information from scratch.

CHOOSING A PHR VENDOR

Personal health records may have a number of important advantages; however, consumers are well advised to consider the issue carefully prior to proceeding and establishing a PHR with a third party, especially one that is hosted online. Personal health records are not considered legal medical records and are not subject to many of the legal protections currently in force. While vendors of PHRs will have breach-notification obligations, they will not be subject to the same requirements as your health care provider with respect to the privacy and security of your medical information. While many people elect to sign up for PHRs because of the convenience and control afforded, using a vendor with inadequate protections can do far more harm than good.

Before selecting a personal health record vendor to manage your medical records, you should investigate that vendor thoroughly. Table 4.1 summarizes a number of key questions to ask before signing up with a PHR vendor.

TABLE 4.1
Investigating a Prospective PHR Vendor

Key Questions to Ask Your PHR Vendor

- Does the vendor have any ownership interest in your information?
- Does the vendor have the right to use your information for any purpose other than providing services to you?
- Can the vendor share your information with any third parties?
  - If so, under what conditions and for what purposes?
  - Do you have any right to opt out of the sharing?
  - Will you receive notice of the sharing?
  - Does the company mine data for any purpose?
- Where are the company's databases located?
- What physical, technical, and administrative measures does it employ to protect the security of your information?
- What disaster recovery policies and procedures does the company have in place?
- Has the vendor suffered security breaches in the past?
- How do you authorize others to access your records?
  - How can you revoke authorization?
- Can you get your full records back upon the termination of your agreement with them?
- Do they retain any of your information after the termination of your agreement?
  - If so, for what purpose and for how long?
- Do they track to whom your information is disclosed, and will they report that to you?

TIPS ON USING A PHR

To maximize the benefits of your PHR, you should include detailed information within it and ensure that you update it regularly to address changes in your health. The following is a list of information that you may wish to include in your PHR.

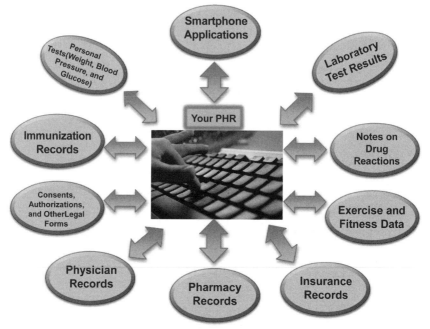

Figure 4.1   Your Personal Health Record (PHR)

Day-to-Day Information

- Personal identification, including name and birth date
- Any information you want to include about your health—such as your exercise regimen, any herbal medications you may take, and any counseling you may receive
- Dietary practices, such as whether you are vegetarian, or on a temporary diet, especially if changes in your diet have produced changes in your health in the past

General Medical Information

- Names, addresses, and phone numbers of your physician, dentist, and specialists
- Health insurance information
- A list and dates of significant illnesses and surgical procedures
- Current medications and dosages
- Immunizations and their dates
- Allergies or sensitivities to drugs or materials, such as latex

Specific Medical Information

- Important events, dates, and hereditary conditions in your family history
- Results from a recent physical examination

- Opinions of specialists
- Important tests results; eye and dental records
- Correspondence between you and your provider(s)
- Current educational materials (or appropriate Web links) relating to your health

Emergency Information

- People to contact in case of emergency
- Living wills, advance directives, or medical power of attorney
- Organ donor authorization

If you do elect to use a PHR, there are steps that you can and should take to increase the likelihood that the privacy and security of your medical records will be maintained.

Perform due diligence in selecting your PHR provider: The prior section on choosing a PHR vendor identified some key questions to explore prior to committing to a particular PHR vendor. Even though many PHR vendors will not charge users a fee, establishing a PHR requires time and effort, and thus some level of commitment. In addition, once information is shared with the provider, you may not have complete control over it. Accordingly, it is best to investigate the provider thoroughly beforehand.

Maintain the security of all hard copies: Whether you decide to implement your own paper-based PHR or an electronic PHR, odds are you will have some paper-based documents containing medical information in your possession. Paper-based PHRs can be challenging, because while you want to keep the records secure from unauthorized access, you also want them handy and accessible. While storing your records in a safe deposit box may reduce the odds that the records will be accessed without authorization, it also reduces the ease with which you can access them. On the other hand, simply storing them in a file folder in a home office will not be very secure. For many, the best solution may be storage in a home-based fireproof safe. Whatever solution is implemented, you should use it consistently, making sure all new records and copies are promptly filed away safely. When records are discarded, they should be destroyed through shredding or other permanent disposal means.

Be secure on the Internet: When storing a PHR electronically, you need to be concerned not only about the providers' security, but also about the security of your own system and network. While accessing your PHR via the Internet can be very convenient, it does entail a number of risks. Many of these risks can be managed through relatively simple techniques that are advisable for the protection of all sensitive information online. For example,

TABLE 4.2
Leading PHR Providers

Name and URL	Fees to End User[1]	Brief Description of Services
Microsoft HealthVault http://www.healthvault.com	None to end-user consumer.	HealthVault provides end-users a means for storing health information from a number of sources in one location. HealthVault has relationships with many third parties (including doctors, hospitals, employers, pharmacies, insurance providers, and manufacturers of health devices) so that users can add information held by those third parties to HealthVault.
Google Health http://www.google.com/health	None to end-user consumer; however, Google Health also provides consumers with access to products and services of other third parties, some of which may charge fees.	Google Health offers a single location to consolidate and store your medical records and personal health information. You can also use Google Health to access a host of online services and tools, from a variety of third-party companies that can help you better manage your care.
Revolution Health http://www.revolutionhealth.com	None to end-user consumer.	Revolution Health keeps track of your medical history, allergies, doctors, and hospitals. Use this to prepare for a doctor visit, create emergency information sheets, or prepare health information when you travel. There is also a public profile that serves as an introduction to the Revolution Health community. It can be used to reach out to others and find people with similar conditions.
Records For Living HealthFrame http://www.recordsforliving.com	Fee service, $39.95 download.	Records For Living has released HealthFrame as a solution to personal health management. They provide professional service to its health provider partners to support the improved exchange of medical record information to their patients.

MyMedicalRecords http://www.mymedicalrecords.com	Fee service, $9.95/month or $99.95/year for up to a family of ten.	MyMedicalRecords.com (MMR) provides consumers with a virtual (online) document and image-management system where they can securely and confidentially store and access their personal health and other information in a simple and easy to use manner. Users then can access their important medical and personal health information, 24/7 from any Internet-connected computer.
Dossia http://www.dossia.org	Not currently available to individuals.	Dossia is a non-profit group comprised of Fortune 500 companies. Dossia aggregates users' health information into one convenient and safe Web-based platform. From this platform, users are not only able to utilize their data, but also have access to personalized health tools that help them improve their health, manage their health conditions, and navigate the health care system.
MyHIN http://www.myhin.org	Fee service.	MyHIN is an online personal health record for individuals living with hydrocephalus.
MyHealtheVet http://www.myhealth.va.gov	None to end-user consumers. Only available to veterans.	My HealtheVet is a free, online personal health record that empowers veterans to become informed partners in their health care. Veterans can access trusted, secure, and current health and benefits information as well as record, track, and store important health and military history information at their convenience. Veterans who are enrolled in a VA facility can refill their VA prescriptions.

(*Continued*)

TABLE 4.2 *(Continued)*

MyMediList http://www.mymedilist.org	None to end-user consumer.	MyMediList is an easy to use, free personal record of your medications and allergies. This electronic medication record is created, modified, and controlled by the patient. Using MyMediList, you can send information to your physician and receive updates from your physician securely.
MyWebMD https://healthmanager.webmd.com	None to end-user consumer.	The personal health manager includes a comprehensive set of health risk assessments, goal-setting, and tracking tools for monitoring progress and results; a personal health record; secure messaging and targeted reminders; lifestyle-improvement programs; accurate, clinically reviewed health information references for any health or medical question; and decision support for understanding the risks and benefits of medical procedures and treatment options.
NoMoreClipboard.com http://www.nomoreclipboard.com	None to end-user consumer	With NoMoreClipboard, you can compile and manage family medical records, and send those records to your physician right from NoMoreClipboard before your next medical appointment.
Telemedical http://www.telemedical.com	None to end-user consumer; however, providers may charge a fee through the use of the site.	Telemedical's PHR module enables online entry of a consumer's lifetime health record. The data is stored in any ODBC-compliant relational database and can be interfaced with existing physician-centric computerized medical record systems. It is a useful tool for health care providers who would like to allow patients to become the primary caregiver.

| MiVIA
http://www.mivia.org | None to end-user consumer. | MiVIA is an online personal health record system where you are able to share your health information with your doctors and other health care providers. A patient photo is required in case of an emergency or if a doctor or clinic is not sure of the name in its files. |
| WorldHealthRecord
http://www.worldhealthrecord.com | None to end-user consumer. | The WorldHealthRecord is a free online personal health record managed and created by you. It contains all of your important health information, which you own and control. |

[1] Be sure to check with the PHR provider for current fee information and services offerings.

maintain the privacy of your usernames and passwords and avoid using ones that could be easy for hackers to crack. This likely sounds as if it were very obvious advice. However, studies show that people continue to use passwords that do not offer them much security.[43]

Controlling access to your PHR: Control who has access to your PHR, limiting it to one or two trusted individuals who can access it in the event of an emergency or an accident in which you are incapacitated.

Update your PHR: The value of your PHR is dependent upon the information that you maintain within it. The most valuable PHRs will be those that are complete and up-to-date. In fact, an incomplete or outdated PHR may be more harmful than useful. If you do elect to maintain a PHR for yourself and/or your family, you should commit to ensure that it remains up-to-date. Here are some suggestions for doing so:

- Review your PHR before each doctor visit.
- Update your PHR promptly after visiting your doctor and/or receiving new health information, such as lab results.
- Maintain hard copies of relevant information (health records, receipts, and other documents).

CONCLUSION

PHRs can be very helpful for the management of your health and medical care. However, as discussed in this chapter, they are not without their risks. Anyone contemplating the possible use of PHRs as vehicles for storing personal health information should research the issues carefully before uploading any information.

Chapter 5 will discuss health privacy at work. There are a surprising number of instances in which your employer may have access to certain details of your health information. Accordingly, it is important to understand the ways in which your employer may and make not use your information. This chapter will also offer guidance on protecting your health privacy in the workplace.

5

Your Health Privacy at Work

INTRODUCTION

At first glance, it may not seem that your employer would be closely involved with your health and/or the privacy of your medical information. As the following scenarios illustrate, however, medical privacy issues can and do arise in the workplace:

You receive a frantic call from your wife, Jane. Between sobs, she explains that she has lost the job she has held for over 15 years. You are immediately confused and taken aback. Your wife has always been very devoted to her job, frequently arriving early and staying late. Your surprise grows as your wife explains that she was fired for failing a surprise drug test conducted at work that day. Now you are completely speechless. To your knowledge, your wife never touched an illegal drug in her life. Slowly, she explains that the drug in question was nicotine. As part of a corporate wellness program, her employer now bans the use of tobacco products by employees and, after being found with nicotine in her system, your wife was immediately fired.

After your best friend leaves you an irate message complaining about your Facebook page, it dawns on you that you have made an epic mistake by posting pictures of your recent rock-climbing trip together. Your friend has been out of work on disability for a back injury, and after a co-worker saw his climbing pictures on your Web page, the co-worker reported him to his supervisor. Now your friend is facing termination and possible legal consequences.

As an employee in a large chain store, you have enjoyed a 20 percent discount on store purchases. One day, however, you receive a communication from your employer advising that you can be eligible for a higher discount (up to 30 percent) if you agree not to smoke, maintain a low cholesterol level, and have an acceptable body mass index, all as confirmed by employer-provided health screenings. You are interested in the higher discount but are wary about submitting to such health screenings, which you consider an intrusive invasion of your privacy. You also question whether such a program might be discriminatory against colleagues who may not be able to fit the established criteria for one reason or another.

These scenarios, while startling, are not far-fetched. In fact, they are based on actual cases. While most may think medical privacy involves only health care providers and insurers, there are a number of situations in which your employer can have access to information concerning your health and, for the most part, employers will not be subject to the same strict medical privacy rules to which your medical provider will be subject.

Furthermore, as will be discussed in this chapter, risks to medical privacy at work are likely to continue to grow as employers, faced with continuously rising health care costs, seek out new ways to ensure that they have healthy, productive workers who will not cost a lot to insure. Although much of 2009 was focused on efforts to pass comprehensive health care reform, at the time of this writing, the full impact of the Patient Protection and Affordable Care Act[1] (PPACA) on health care costs was not yet clear and, in fact, may not be for some time. Still, there are plenty of critics who contend that the new controversial legislation will not lead to reduced costs for employers.[2] If these predictions hold true (and again, even if they don't),[3] then you can bet that employers will continue to seek out new ways to reduce health care costs.

In light of this very complicated backdrop, this chapter will explore the health privacy issues that impact individuals in connection with the relationships with employers. It will include discussions of issues such as data collection during pre-employment screening and hiring, wellness programs at work, and the disclosure of health-related information in social-networking Web sites and other Web-based forums.

YOUR EMPLOYER'S INTEREST IN YOUR MEDICAL INFORMATION

There are a number of instances in which your employer may have a legitimate interest in obtaining, using, and/or sharing certain information concerning your health. For example, if you suffer an injury at work and need to file for worker's compensation, your employer will require certain information from you and/or your medical providers. The same holds true if you will be taking an extended medical leave. With limitations (to be discussed later on in this chapter), an employer may also request certain medical information as part of an employee background check.

Employers may also need to collect or authorize a designated third party to collect certain information about your health in order to administer wellness programs. Increasingly, employers have a strong desire to ensure that their workforces are fit and healthy and are developing new programs to encourage employees to adopt behaviors that are likely to have a positive impact on their health. These various initiatives will be discussed in more detail later in this chapter in the section entitled "Wellness Programs at Work." In designing, implementing, and monitoring the effects of these programs, employers are often likely to require certain medical information from their employees. For example, if a program provides incentives for achieving certain cholesterol or blood pressure levels, the employer may require participating employees to submit to screenings or otherwise provide data regarding their cholesterol and/or blood pressure levels. Again, as will be discussed, there are limitations on the information that an employer can request and how they can use medical information.

While the preceding paragraphs describe some of the main ways in which your employer can access your medical data, they are not the only ways. For example, your employer may access medical information that you voluntarily disclose to the employer, that you share with third parties who then disclose the information to your employer, and/or that you disclose in public forums, such as Web sites. An employer may also have access to your medical information in a range of other scenarios, such as when your employer must report information to government agencies in the event of a public health crisis or when you are involved in litigation with your employer concerning an illness or injury.

The key thing to remember when you are making voluntary disclosures of medical information to your employer (or public disclosures that may make their way back to your current employer or a prospective employer) is that your employer is not under the same legal obligations and professional duties to keep your medical information confidential as your health care provider is under. Moreover, when you give medical information to your health care provider, typically the primary reason that you do is so that your provider can give you appropriate medical care. Obviously, this is not the case when medical information is provided to and/or collected by your employer. Accordingly, it will usually be in your best interest to limit the health information that you share with your employer.

HIPAA AND YOUR EMPLOYER

For most employees, the impact of HIPAA on workplace privacy is rather limited. As discussed, HIPAA's Privacy and Security Rules apply only to covered entities and their business associates. The rules do not extend more generally to all private-sector companies. The HIPAA Privacy Rule does not protect the privacy of your work records, even if those records contain health-related information. However, the HIPAA Privacy Rule does, of course, control how a covered entity, such as a health plan or health care provider, discloses protected health information to an employer.

The situation becomes a bit more complex if you are working for a covered entity that is subject to HIPAA. An individual working for a hospital, for example, may assume that as a covered entity, their employer is obliged to comply with the HIPAA Privacy Rule and the HIPAA Security Rule in connection with all employees' medical information. However, this assumption would be incorrect. The HIPAA Privacy Rule protects your medical and health plan records if you are a patient of the provider or a member of the health plan, but it does not apply to your employment records if you are an employee of such an entity.

Given the HIPAA Privacy Rule's limited scope, it generally will not prevent your supervisor, human resources director, or other administrators within your company from asking you for certain health-related information. For example, if you are out sick, an employer may request a doctor's note, and the note may result in your employer having access to certain information about your health. An employer may request information about your health to administer sick leave, workers' compensation, wellness programs, or health insurance.

Generally, a covered entity must have your authorization to disclose information to your employer, unless other laws require them to comply with the employer's request. HIPAA does not, however, prevent your employer from asking questions of you directly. In other words, from a legal perspective, there is an enormous and very important difference between an employer asking you for medical data and an employer contacting your doctor directly to get information. The HIPAA Privacy Rule applies to disclosures made by your health care provider, but not to the questions of your employer—and your answers. Accordingly, to maximize the protection of your health privacy at work, be cautious about sharing medical information with your employer and provide only the minimum amount necessary. Also, as discussed earlier in Chapter 2, you must be very careful about signing authorizations and, in particular, any broad or blanket authorizations you may be asked to execute. Review all authorization forms very carefully and make sure that you understand their terms before signing. As always, if you have any questions or doubts about what you are being asked to sign, you should get appropriate legal advice.

PRE-EMPLOYMENT SCREENING AND HIRING

An employer's interest in collecting health information about you may be piqued as early on as the recruitment process. Employers may wish to obtain certain information about a prospective employee's medical status for a variety of reasons, such as to ensure that the employee can perform the job tasks for which they are being recruited, to minimize the risks of hiring an employee who will miss a lot of work due to illness, and to reduce the likelihood that the employee will be costly to insure. There are, however, legal limitations on what an employer can acquire, and they vary depending on the stage of the hiring process.

The key legislation here is the Americans with Disabilities Act (ADA).[4] Notwithstanding its name, the reach of the ADA is not limited to disabled employees. In fact, the law has important implications in the recruitment and employee of all employees—disabled or not. The ADA affects the content of advertisements for employment, job applications, interviews, and post-offer medical examinations.[5]

Under the ADA, employers cannot ask job applicants medical-related questions before a job offer is made.[6] In practice, this means that an employer generally cannot include on job applications or in interviews any questions that are likely to elicit information about a disability. For instance, a prospective employer could not ask a job applicant if she has a physical or mental impairment. It also means that an employer could not ask about past medical conditions, such as if the applicant had previously filed a workers' compensation claim. Before an offer is made, a prospective employer may only ask about the applicant's ability to perform job-related functions.[7]

Although the ADA's prohibitions apply to medical inquiries concerning whether an applicant is "an individual with a disability or as to the nature or severity of such disability,"[8] documents produced by the Equal Employment Opportunity Commission (EEOC) suggest that it interprets the applicable ADA provisions as prohibiting virtually all health-related inquiries.[9]

In its manual on the ADA, the EEOC indentifies a list of questions that employers are advised to refrain from asking prospective employees, such as:[10]

- Have you ever been treated by a psychiatrist or psychologist? If so, for what condition?
- Have you had a major illness in the last five years?
- Have you ever been hospitalized, and if so, for what condition?
- How many days were you absent from work because of illness last year?

These questions are illustrative of the types of prohibited questions you may encounter when seeking employment. They do not constitute an all-inclusive list of restricted questions. When seeking employment, you should always be wary of any health-related questions that appear on a job application or are asked in an interview. Prior to seeking and/or applying for a new job, ensure that you are aware of your rights and the restrictions that are imposed upon prospective employers.

The scope of permitted health-related inquiries an employer may make changes once a bona fide offer of employment has been made (and then, as will be discussed, changes again once the applicant becomes an actual employee). Under the ADA, once an employer has extended a job offer to an applicant, the employer may require the applicant to submit to a medical exam prior to commencing work, but only if the employer requires all other entering employees in the same job category to take the same exam.[11] This requirement has an important rationale—the ADA prohibits employers from forcing applicants to undergo any medical examination until after a valid job offer is made to ensure that employers don't consider an applicant's disability when determining whether or not to extend an offer of employment. The ADA also imposes confidentiality obligations with respect to the information that is collected by the employer in conducting the exam. Specifically, the ADA requires that the information be "collected and maintained on separate forms also to boost confidentiality and in separate medical files."[12] This is important, because again, employers are not subject to the HIPAA Security Rule, nor, obviously, are they subject to the professional duties of confidentiality to which your medical providers are bound.

Once a bona fide job offer has been extended, in addition to being able to conduct the medical exam, the employer may ask medically-related questions as long as the procedural and confidentiality requirements of the ADA are met. While employers can collect a wide array of medical information once a job offer is made, they can use only the portions of the information that relate to job performance when making employment decisions.

Different rules apply with respect to inquires that may be made of existing employees. Under the ADA, employers are permitted to ask about employees' abilities to perform job functions and may subject employees to medical inquiries or exams, but only those that are "shown to be job-related and consistent with business necessity."[13] Also, it is important to note that regulators have attempted to limit the ability of employers to collect the restricted information through other means. According to the EEOC employers may not bypass the limitations of the ADA by collecting information indirectly, such as by gathering information about the employee's medical status from family, friends, co-workers, or doctors, or by searching an employee's belongings.[14]

WELLNESS PROGRAMS AT WORK

Introduction to Employer-Sponsored Wellness Programs

As is evidenced by all the attention that has been devoted to health care reform, the cost of health care is a major problem in the United States. Spending on health care, already astronomically high, is projected to continue to rise over the next 10 years, reaching $4 trillion in 2015, a figure set to equal 20 percent of the nation's gross domestic product.[15] Not surprisingly, the cost of health care is a major concern for many employers, who often have to bear at least some of the costs of insuring employees. The data on this point are painfully clear. Consider, for example, that between 1999 and 2008, the cost of family health insurance premiums increased an astonishing 119 percent.[16]

Many employers concerned about productivity, as well as the rising costs of health care, have begun to explore a wide range of employee wellness programs. Simply speaking, wellness programs are organized and coordinated programs that have the goal of enhancing the physical, mental, and emotional status of individuals. Many wellness programs are designed to influence employees to engage in healthy behaviors in the hope that improved health behaviors will lead to healthier employees, reductions in absenteeism, improved employee morale, and increased productivity, all while also helping to reign in health insurance costs.

Employers may offer incentives to spur employee participation in these programs, and some are even seeking ways to require participation. Today's programs have moved far beyond mere rebates for gym memberships, with employers offering a variety of creative programs, including:

- Disease and case-management programs
- Subsidized healthy meals at work
- Time to exercise during the workday
- Incentive programs that reward desirable health behaviors
- Online health-management tools and/or hotlines staffed with nurses or other medical professionals

The data on the prevalence of wellness programs is not 100 percent clear, with most figures relying upon self-reported responses to surveys that may involve differing definitions of wellness programs. For example, while one 2008 survey reported that more that 70 percent of employers offered some form of wellness program,[17] a March 2009 nationwide survey conducted by the John J. Heldrich Center for Workforce Development at Rutgers University revealed that 38 percent of employers provide some kind of wellness programs, with offerings regarding fitness and stress management the most prevalent.[18]

Among employees, there seem to be some mixed feelings about wellness programs at work. For instance, while the Rutgers study revealed that there is strong support among workers for wellness programs, it also showed that real concerns about the privacy implications of such programs.[19]

The approaches employers take in designing their programs vary considerably. The next section will examine in further detail the two main types of programs: incentive-based participatory programs and those that reward the achievement of a particular goal.

Types of Wellness Programs

Participatory Versus Rewards-Based Programs

Many wellness programs provide incentives for participation rather than rewarding the achievement of a particular health-related target or standard. Below are some examples of participatory wellness programs:

- Programs that reimburse gym memberships
- Programs that provide incentives to participate in blood pressure, cholesterol or similar screenings, where the incentive is paid, regardless of the outcome (i.e., whether cholesterol levels and/or blood pressure has gone down or up)
- Programs that provide incentives or rewards for attending educational seminars, such as healthy eating or stress-management classes
- Programs that provide incentives for participating in smoking cessation or weight loss programs, irrespective of outcome

Because these types of programs reward participation as opposed to the achievement of certain goals, they are the least likely to raise legal and regulatory concerns. In particular, as will be discussed in greater detail in the section of this chapter titled under "Key Legal Issues," participatory wellness programs are not likely to be considered discriminatory under HIPAA's non-discrimination rules.

As employers continue to seek out the most effective means of improving employee health and reducing employee health care costs, some are looking beyond programs that reward employees for the mere participation in a particular program and are instead seeking to develop wellness programs that will reward the attainment of specific health and/or fitness goals. There are a number of different types of these programs; some examples are set forth below:

- Programs that provide incentives to individuals who participate in blood pressure and/or cholesterol screening programs if certain targets are achieved.
- Smoking cessation and/or weight loss programs that provide incentives if the employee ceases smoking and/or sheds weight, as applicable.
- Programs that reimburse gym membership fees only if certain fitness and/or weight-loss goals are achieved.

Programs that reward the achievement of certain goals, while attractive to some employers, can also be problematic due to the existing legal and regulatory framework. These issues will be discussed further in the next section on key legal issues.

Examples of Programs

Although workplace wellness programs are increasing in popularity, a few really stand out as examples that are worthy of highlight. Scotts Miracle Grow

(Scotts)[20] is particularly notable, as the company has implemented an especially comprehensive wellness program that may also be considered as rather aggressive in its efforts to reduce health care costs and improve health and fitness among employees. The company offers its employees in-depth health assessments, and while they are not required to participate in the assessments, those who do participate do not pay additional monthly insurance premiums.[21] An outside health-management company examines the results of the health assessment as well as the employee's family and medical history and cross-references this information with insurance claim data.[22] Employees are then assigned a risk level, and those who are identified as moderate or high risk are assigned a health coach who then develops an action plan for the employee.[23] Failure to comply with the assigned plan can result in additional premiums.[24] Scotts also encourages preventative care by offering employees access to a free on-site health clinic and fitness center.[25]

Scotts also has a very restrictive tobacco policy. The company is totally tobacco-free—employees are not only prohibited from using tobacco at work, they are also prohibited from using tobacco at home or elsewhere off working hours.[26] The company's strong anti-tobacco policy has brought it some unwanted attention. After the company reportedly terminated the employment of a new hire whose urine tested positive for nicotine, the employee filed suit against Scotts,[27] alleging a violation of privacy rights under state law, as well as interference with his rights to benefits and wrongful termination.[28]

Scotts is certainly not the only enterprise to focus on tobacco cessation. This is, in fact, a very common attribute of workplace wellness programs, and many companies focused upon improving employee health have adopted strong anti-tobacco programs. In 2004, the president of Weyco, a Michigan insurance consulting firm announced that any employee who tested positive for nicotine would be terminated. The company gave its employees 15 months to quit and offered smoking-cessation assistance.[29] In January 2005, the company began random nicotine testing on its employees.[30] While Weyco's ban was subject to some criticism from civil libertarian and smokers' rights groups,[31] the ban was permissible under Michigan law—the state is one of a minority of states that has not passed a law to preventing employers from firing workers who engage in legal conduct, such as smoking, outside of working hours.

Likewise, in 2007, the Cleveland Clinic added nicotine testing to its pre-employment tests, with positive tests resulting in rejection of employment.[32] However, the clinic also offers smoking-cessation services to applicants who are rejected for positive nicotine tests. Prior to the anti-tobacco policy, the clinic had already taken strides toward improving the health and wellness of employees—and visitors—by removing sugar-sweetened beverages from its vending machines and trans fats from its cafeterias.[33]

Although anti-tobacco initiatives such as those described above may be considered quite popular among health care advocates and those who seek to rein in health care costs, as will be discussed in the section titled "The Problem of Monitoring and/or Regulating Off-Duty Conduct," due to state laws that limit how far an employer can go in regulating the legal behavior of employees outside of working hours, these kinds of initiatives will not be possible in all states.

Key Legal Issues

Employers need to be concerned with a number of laws when designing and administering their wellness programs. At the federal level, employers need to be most concerned about the HIPAA non-discrimination rules,[34] the ADA, and the Genetic Information Non-Discrimination Act (GINA).[35] Of course, state laws can also impact wellness programs. This is particularly the case with respect to state laws concerning privacy rights and the rights of employees to engage in lawful conduct outside of working hours. These issues, which are increasing important in connection with wellness programs at work, will be discussed. However, we will first examine the key federal laws applicable to employer-sponsored wellness programs and how they regulate the implementation and administration of wellness programs at work.

HIPAA Non-Discrimination Rules

HIPAA's non-discrimination rules have important implications for wellness programs. While must of this book has focused upon HIPAA's Privacy Rule and Security Rule, HIPAA goes far beyond regulating the privacy and security of health information. Significant to the discussion of workplace wellness programs are HIPAA's non-discrimination rules. HIPAA requires group health insurance plans to offer enrollment in the plan to all eligible group members regardless of any individual's health status and prohibits the group plan from charging any plan member a higher premium than others in the group because of a "health factor."[36] A health factor, in turn, is any of the following: (1) health status; (2) medical condition (including both physical and mental illnesses); (3) claims experience; (4) receipt of health care; (5) medical history; (6) genetic information; (7) events of insurability (including conditions arising out of acts of domestic violence); and/or (8) disability.[37] Accordingly, generally speaking, if a group health plan offers insurance to a group of employees at a particular company, the plan could not go through the medical histories of the employees and charge different premiums to employees based upon their medical histories.

These non-discrimination rules are an important part of the rationale for the enactment of HIPAA. When the law was enacted back in 1996, one of its main goals was to prevent a scenario wherein an employee would feel she needed to remain at a particular job because she had a preexisting condition and feared that this preexisting condition would result in a need to pay prohibitively high health insurance premiums at a new employer.

Given the fact that HIPAA prohibits group health plans from charging any plan member a higher premium than other members of the group because of a "health factor," one may question whether workplace wellness programs that provide financial incentives for the achievement of health goals can be permissible. In response to the growing popularity of wellness programs, the government has responded with additional regulations. On December 13, 2006, the Department of Labor, the Department of the Treasury, and the Department of Health and Human Services issued final regulations that set standards for "wellness programs," described as health promotion and disease programs through which an employer may be able to require compliance in order to take advantage of premium discounts and rebates consistent with the non-discrimination rules.[38]

Under the regulations, a group health plan may offer premium discounts, impose surcharges, grant rebates, and otherwise create premium differentials between employees in exchange for adherence to a wellness program.[39] Some programs reimburse employees for attending smoking-cessation classes, whether or not the employee quits, or provide reimbursement for gym memberships, even if the employee's health doesn't improve. But the government regulations really only come into play for programs in which incentives are based on results (i.e., the employee quits smoking or reaches his/her body mass index goal).

If the reward is contingent on results, the following five requirements must be met under the HIPAA regulations to qualify as a wellness program and not be discriminatory.[40] Each of these factors is examined in further detail below.

1. The reward provided to the employee may not exceed 20 percent of the total cost of the employee-only coverage. (Although the PPACA is increasing this to 30 percent).

2. The program must be reasonably designed to promote heath or prevent disease.

3. The program must allow eligible individuals an opportunity to qualify for the award at least annually.

4. The program must be available to similarly situated individuals; if it would be unreasonably difficult or medically inadvisable for an individual to attempt to satisfy the standard, the program must provide a reasonable alternative.

5. All materials describing the key terms of the program must disclose the availability of a reasonable alternative standard or the possibility of obtaining a waiver of the applicable standard.

First, the total reward for all wellness programs must not exceed 20 percent of the cost of employee-only coverage under the related health plan. (Recall that under the PPACA, this figure will be increased to 30 percent). This employee-only cost is determined based on the total amount of employer and employee contributions. However, if in addition to employees, any class of dependents (such as spouses and dependent children) participates in the wellness program, the reward must not exceed 20 percent (soon 30 percent) of the cost of the coverage in which an employee and any dependents are enrolled.[41]

Second, the program must be "reasonably designed" to promote good health or prevent disease. A program satisfies this standard if it: (i) has a reasonable chance of improving the health of or preventing disease in participating individuals and is not overly burdensome; (ii) is not a subterfuge for discriminating based on a health factor; and (iii) is not highly suspect in the method chosen to promote health or prevent disease.[42] The "reasonably designed" standard is intended to be fairly easy to meet. According to the regulations:

There does not need to be a scientific record that the method promotes wellness to satisfy this standard. The standard is intended to allow experimentation in diverse ways of promoting wellness. For example, a plan or issuer could satisfy this standard by providing rewards to individuals who participated in a course of stress management and relaxation techniques. The requirement of reasonableness in this standard prohibits bizarre, extreme, or illegal requirements in a wellness program.[43]

Third, the program must give individuals the opportunity to qualify for the reward at least once per year.[44] This requirement is important because it ensures that programs give individuals the opportunity to improve their health or wellness compliance over time. Otherwise, a program could simply be a cover for rewarding individuals who meet the standard at the time the program is implemented and discriminate on an ongoing basis against those who cannot meet the program's standards.

Fourth, the reward must be available to all similarly situated individuals.[45] More specifically, the program must offer alternatives or grant waivers to those whom it is unreasonably difficult (or inadvisable) to meet the wellness program standard due to a medical condition. It may be difficult for employers to determine what might be a reasonable alternative for any given employee. Accordingly, it is important to note that employers can seek the advice of medical professionals when devising reasonable alternatives. Also, employers may seek verification (e.g., a statement from a participant's physician) that a person can't participate due to a health factor.[46] When it comes to smoking, for example, regulations and guidance from the Department of Labor indicate that medical evidence suggests nicotine addiction is likely a "health factor."[47] So if a wellness program offers a reward for those who quit smoking, a reasonable alternative must also be provided.

In other words, if an employee with a nicotine addiction can't seem to quit, an employer must offer another way to obtain the reward, such as smoking-cessation classes. Even if the employee attends the classes but doesn't quit smoking, she's not penalized because of her addiction.

An employer may require an employee to obtain certification from her physician that she is addicted to nicotine before the employer would be required to provide an alternative.[48] In other words, if the employee was not willing to go to his or her physician to certify nicotine addiction, the employer could deny the reward without offering an alternative. This strategy could have two potential positive effects: (1) it would require employees to have an honest conversation with their physician about their tobacco use; and/or (2) it would discourage individuals who might abuse the program because they might not want to return to their physician annually to get recertified. Of course, this might also discourage those who might not be willing to go to their physician but who might be willing to enroll in a smoking-cessation program.

Finally, plan materials must disclose the availability of a reasonable alternative standard or the possibility of a waiver of the wellness program standard.[49] Plan materials are not required to detail specific alternatives; it is sufficient to disclose that some reasonable alternative will be made available. The regulations provide model language that may be used to satisfy this disclosure requirement, as set forth below:

Sample Disclosure Language:

If it is unreasonably difficult due to a medical condition for you to achieve the standards for the reward under this program, or if it is medically inadvisable for you to attempt to achieve the standards for the reward under this program, call us at [insert telephone number] and we will work with you to develop another way to qualify for this reward.[50]

Americans with Disabilities Act

The ADA also has implications for wellness programs. To function as intended, most wellness programs will require employees to complete medical questionnaires and undergo medical examinations. However, the ADA dictates that once someone is employed, the employer may make only disability-related inquiries and require medical examinations if they are "job-related and consistent with business necessity."[51]

While wellness programs may be beneficial to both employer and employees, they have never been interpreted in any official guidance or case law as satisfying the "job-related and consistent with business necessity" requirement under the ADA. Therefore, any wellness program that makes disability-related inquiries or requires medical examinations violates the ADA, unless it falls within the exception for "voluntary wellness programs."[52] Under this exception, the employer does not have to show that disability-related inquiries or medical examinations are job-related and consistent with business necessity, as long as records are kept confidential and separate from personnel records. Voluntary wellness programs can include such medical examinations as blood pressure screening, cholesterol testing, glaucoma testing, and cancer-detection screening.[53]

The ADA states that an employer "may conduct voluntary medical examinations, including voluntary medical histories, which are part of an employee health program available to employees at that work site" even though such examinations are not job-related and consistent with business necessity.[54] The applicable regulations repeat this provision almost verbatim without providing any further interpretation of what it means to conduct a "voluntary" medical examination.[55] However, in guidance, the EEOC has stated that a "wellness program is 'voluntary' as long as an employer neither requires participation nor penalizes employees who do not participate."[56] The EEOC addressed the issue on two separate occasions in 2009, stating its view that if an employee's eligibility in an employer's health care plan is conditioned upon completion of a health risk assessment that makes disability-related inquiries and requires medical examinations, such health risk assessment does not qualify as a "voluntary wellness program," and therefore violates the ADA.

On March 6, 2009, the EEOC issued an Informal Discussion Letter[57] (the "March Letter") in which it provided its informal opinion as to whether certain wellness programs were in fact "voluntary" for purposes of the exception. The employer that had sought the opinion of the EEOC was a county that required county employees to participate in a health risk assessment as a condition for participating in its health insurance plan. The health risk assessment included answering a short, health-related questionnaire, taking a blood pressure test, and providing blood for use in a blood panel screen. Results from the assessment went directly and exclusively to the employee, and the county only received information in the aggregate.

In the March Letter, the EEOC first stated that requiring completion of the health risk assessment "does not appear to be job-related and consistent with business necessity, and therefore would violate the ADA."[58] The March Letter then discussed the exception provided when disability-related inquiries and medical examinations are part of a voluntary wellness program. On this point, the letter stated:

A wellness program is voluntary if employees are neither required to participate nor penalized for non-participation. In this instance, however, an employee's decision not to participate in the health risk assessment results in the loss of the opportunity to obtain health coverage through the employer's plan. Thus, even if the health risk assessment could be considered part of a wellness program, the program would not be voluntary, because individuals who do not participate in the assessment are denied a benefit (i.e., penalized for non-participation) as compared to employees who participate in the assessment.[59] (Internal citations omitted.)

On August 10, 2009, the EEOC issued a second Informal Discussion Letter (the "August Letter") that further clarifies the meaning of "voluntary" in connection with such employer programs.[60] The employer seeking this discussion letter from the EEOC had required its employees to complete a health risk assessment containing more than 100 questions in order to receive money from an employer-funded health reimbursement arrangement (but it did not require medical examinations). The EEOC was consistent with the position it took in its earlier discussion letter on this topic. More specifically, the EEOC found that the health risk assessment was not voluntary because employees were penalized for nonparticipation, and thus it concluded that the described program would violate the ADA.[61]

The EEOC did note, however, that only the disability-related inquiries on the health risk assessment appeared to violate the ADA. It specifically noted that questions about lifestyle, such as whether an employee sees a personal doctor for routine care or has a health care directive, and questions relating to personal nutrition and exercise are not likely, in its view, to elicit information about a disability, and are therefore not subject to the ADA's restrictions.[62] Thus, this August Letter is helpful not only for its guidance on what is and what is not voluntary (e.g., penalizing employees who do not participate makes the program non-voluntary), but it also offers guidance on the types of assessment questions that are likely to trigger ADA concerns (as well as those that may not).

Genetic Non-Discrimination Act (GINA)

Wellness programs must also comply with the GINA.[63] Some employers may wish to use genetic information to assist employees to help them manage their health. For example, for some disorders, once genetic testing reveals a predisposition to the disorder, lifestyle changes may help an individual to delay the onset of the disorder or mitigate the effects of it. However, under new regulations issued on October 7, 2009,[64] wellness programs that request genetic information, including family medical history, violate GINA, whether or not rewards are based on the outcome of the health risk assessment.

GINA concerns "genetic information," which is defined broadly to mean information about: (a) the individual's genetic tests; (b) the genetic tests of his or her family members; (c) the manifestation of a disease or disorder in family members of the individual; or (d) any request for, or receipt of, genetic services, or participation in clinical research that includes genetic services by the individual or any of his or her family members.[65] This definition relies on a few other definitions, which are worthy of note. First, a "genetic test" is "an analysis of human DNA, RNA, chromosomes, proteins, or metabolites, that detects genotypes, mutations, or chromosomal changes."[66] Also, "underwriting purposes" are defined to include, among others, rules for eligibility, computation of premiums, application of pre-existing condition exclusions, and "other activities related to the creation, renewal, or replacement of a contract of health insurance or health benefits."[67]

GINA prohibits group health plans and any wellness programs the plans offer from doing three main things with respect to genetic information:

- Adjusting premiums or contribution amounts of individuals in a group coverage plan on the basis of genetic information;
- Requesting or requiring an individual or family member of the individual to undergo a genetic test; and
- Collecting genetic information for underwriting purposes, and also collecting genetic information with respect to an individual prior to enrollment.[68]

Of special concern to many employers is how GINA will impact their implementation of wellness programs and health risk assessments, since many assessments ask a wide range of health-related questions. These assessments often including questions about family health history, which is considered "genetic information" under GINA. Under GINA, a group health plan may not collect genetic information for underwriting purposes, nor may it collect genetic information with respect to any individual prior to that individual's effective date of coverage under the plan.[69] The new interim regulations set forth numerous examples of how this prohibition impacts health risk assessments. In sum, if an assessment seeks information about an individual's family history, *and* if completing the health risk assessment will result in a premium reduction, then the group health plan is impermissibly collecting genetic information for underwriting purposes. On the other hand, if completing the assessment has *no* impact on premiums (or any other underwriting purpose) and its completion is not required prior to, or as a condition for, enrollment in the group health plan, then GINA would not prohibit the collection of data concerning the employee's family history.[70]

Privacy Matters

Wellness programs can also give rise to privacy issues—under HIPAA and beyond. As has been discussed, the HIPAA Privacy Rule governs how a health plan may use and disclose personal health information (PHI). The information provided via a wellness program should be treated like any other PHI received by a health plan and should be protected under the Privacy Rule.[71]

For example, the information should be used and disclosed only for purposes related to operating the wellness program. This means that access to PHI should be restricted to the people who are administering the program. Similarly, the information should not be used for any employment- or benefit-related decisions. Any use or disclosure of a participant's PHI outside of the program must be disclosed and authorized by the participant. All employers who maintain health plans and/or wellness programs should undergo an analysis of their use and disclosure of PHI from the plan or program, have in place a HIPAA compliance program, and consult state law on the uses and disclosures of health information in connection with wellness programs.

Additionally, employers need to be aware of privacy obligations they may have under the ADA. Even if a wellness program is not subject to HIPAA, it must still comply with the ADA requirement to keep employees' medical information confidential. In general, the ADA requires that any information obtained "regarding the medical condition or history of any employee shall be collected and maintained on separate forms and in separate medical files and be treated as a confidential medical record."[72] Exceptions apply when there is a need to provide accommodations to an employee, when emergency medical care may be required, and in the case of governmental investigations.[73] In the normal course of business, however, an employer needs to have the procedures in place to keep information obtained through its wellness program confidential and completely separate from employee personnel files.

The Problem of Monitoring and/or Regulating Off-Duty Conduct

Some employers wish to take wellness programs a step further by extending certain elements of the programs to an employee's off-duty conduct. Earlier, the discussion of examples of programs demonstrated how certain companies are going beyond prohibiting smoking in the workplace to completely banning all tobacco use by employees, whether done within or outside of working hours. There is clear and sound rationale for the notion of extending wellness program requirements outside of the parameters of the workplace. After all, a workplace wellness program that gets employees to refrain from smoking or eating unhealthy food will only get the employee part of the way to good health if he or she is free to smoke or eat unhealthy foods while off-duty. In fact, the program may not even make a dent in the problem if the employee makes up for the workplace abstinence by wolfing down extra amounts of unhealthy foods or smoking like a chimney when not at work.

Accordingly, many employers that have adopted workplace wellness programs have an interest in monitoring and/or regulating some aspects of their workers' off-duty conduct. This, however, can raise significant legal, business, and ethical issues. From an ethical perspective, these kinds of programs raise potential concerns about lifestyle discrimination. There are real questions about how far employers should rightfully be able to interfere in the private lives of employees. For some lifestyle choices, such as smoking, the links with potential negative health consequences are clear and well established.[74] However, as noted, many employers are extending the reach of their wellness programs beyond smoking and covering issues such as body mass index (BMI), where causal relationships with good health are more tenuous.[75] Additionally, there does seem to be a risk for embarking upon a slippery slope. For instance, while it is true that smoking can be harmful to human health, clearly this is not the only behavior that can have negative health consequences. A wide range of activities, including speeding, engaging in certain adventure sports and other high-risk leisure activities, and failing to follow medical treatment protocols for diagnosed disorders can all lead to employee injuries and illnesses, resulting in high health care costs and employee absenteeism. If, as a society, we are to accept employer involvement in controlling employee behaviors, such as smoking, eating, and physical exercise, will control of other aspects of legal off-duty conduct be much further down the road?

The regulation of off-duty conduct also raises legal issues. In many states, for example, an employer's efforts to monitor and/or regulate the off-duty legal conduct of employees may not be legal. In fact, at least 30 states and the District of Columbia have enacted laws that prohibit employment discrimination against workers who smoke outside of their place of employment.[76] A smaller but still sizeable number of states restrict employers from prohibiting their employees from using alcohol outside of the workplace. Further, a handful of states (Colorado, North Dakota, California, and New York) have enacted laws that provide for broader protection of a wide range of off-duty conduct.[77]

Of course, there are important distinctions between off-duty legal conduct and off-duty illegal conduct. Let's go back to Scenario 1, covered earlier. If Jane was residing in a state that prohibited employers from penalizing employees for their off-duty legal conduct, her employer could not have terminated her for having tobacco in her system. The result, however, would have been quite different—even in a state that protects against employer action for legal off-duty conduct—if the substance was cocaine, heroin, or any other illegal drug.

Programs of this nature, while likely to continue to grow in the future, are still often viewed as somewhat controversial. For example, when grocer Whole Foods recently unveiled a program to provide higher employee discounts to employees who agreed to submit to health screenings and maintain certain health standards, the program was viewed with some skepticism and criticism.[78] Previously, all store employees received a 20 percent discount on store purchases. However, the grocery chain recently offered employees the opportunity to sign up for a voluntary program that allowed them to become eligible for discounts of up to 30 percent if they agreed to submit to health screenings, refrained from smoking, and maintained low blood pressure, cholesterol, and body mass index (BMI) rates. While the program can be viewed as a rather innovative way of encouraging better health behaviors, advocates for the overweight condemned it and urged a boycott, contending that the program was discriminatory and rewarded people who were naturally thin.[79]

Accordingly, where the regulation of off-duty legal conduct is permissible under applicable law, employers will still need to analyze whether these kinds of programs will be good for business. This will involve investigating the possible savings the company might generate through the expanded wellness program and comparing it to any losses that it may experience if the wellness program has a negative impact on the ability of the company to recruit the best candidates.

SOCIAL NETWORKING, PRIVACY, AND YOUR EMPLOYER

Although one of the main goals of this book is to outline some of the key external risks to our health privacy, it is also important to understand how our actions—or our failures to act—can make ourselves more vulnerable to privacy violations. It is undeniable that we all have a very important role to play in our own privacy protection, whether in connection with one's employment or just generally. In the current era, people are more inclined than ever to make personal disclosures to huge audiences on social-networking Web sites like Facebook. While many of these sites have sophisticated privacy controls that allow individuals to control what personal information is shared and with whom, these controls are not infallible. Moreover, many of the privacy protections offered by social-networking sites depend on users reading about, understanding, and selecting the controls and preferences that they feel will offer them a robust user experience while also providing sufficient privacy protection. For many Web sites, relying upon default settings will not offer the most privacy protection. Furthermore, even where a user does all in her power to make her own online experience as protective of privacy as possible, she won't be able to effectively control all of the actions of her friends and contacts. Recall, for example, the second scenario at the beginning of this chapter where one person's posting of rock-climbing pictures on a social-networking site led to seriously negative consequences for a friend who was included in those photos but who did not play a role in the posting of those photographs.

Some individuals facing certain health challenges are embracing social networking as a means of communicating with family and friends about their health status, for finding support and encouragement from similarly afflicted individuals, and for exchanging information about new treatments, drugs, and other therapies.

There are a number of ways in which people may elect to share health-related information online. On one side of the spectrum, an individual may disclose that she is suffering from a particular ailment by updating her Facebook status to reflect that she is in the hospital recovering from surgery or is off to get another drug infusion. On the other side of the spectrum, an individual may elect to participate in a Web site that has been established to serve as an online community for those facing particular health challenges. There are a number of Web sites that are devoted to particular ailments. For example, dLife.com is an online community for people with diabetes and KnowCancer.com is a well-known resource dedicated to helping people suffering from various forms of cancer. Other sites, such as HealingWell.com, focus on a number of different ailments. The Internet has become a tremendous resource and support network for individuals with various health concerns. Many Web sites offer forums through which participants may disclose more detailed information, including experiences with certain treatments and details of surgeries and medications. Participants may also ask questions and respond to questions posted by other users.

People using these online communities may often elect to do so without disclosing any of their personal data. They may, for example, register with a user name that does not define them (such as, for example, HockeyFan728). However, participants in these online health communities often post pictures and/or share other personal information that may make them identifiable. Moreover, even when an individual feels that he is using an online community on a private, confidential, and anonymous basis, he may end up revealing more than he may have intended to or believed he has.

As with PHRs, privacy and security for social-networking participants also hinges on the policies and procedures of the Web site being used. Even if an individual intends on using a particular online service in a private and confidential manner, those plans may fail if the Web site does not comply with its privacy commitments and/or maintain adequate security.

The potential problems of revealing information online through social networks is highlighted in Scenario 2 at the beginning of this chapter. (As noted, this scenario highlights the potential risks of disclosures made by others, including your close friends and contacts.) The potential problems of personal disclosures online is further emphasized by a recent case involving a 29-year-old IBM employee who was on disability leave because she claimed she was too depressed to work. During that time, the woman went to a birthday party and on a family vacation. After the events, she innocently posted the pictures to her Facebook account. She claimed her doctor told her that the vacation would do her good, but her insurance company did not agree. After becoming aware of the online photos, the insurer stopped making disability payments to her. As a result, the woman has been forced to sell her house after failing to meet her mortgage payments, and has suffered damage to her credit and reputation. She argued that the happiness in the pictures was fleeting and does not reflect her normal day-to-day state of mind, and she has filed suit to recover the lost payments.[80]

While this section has focused on the potential impact of online social network postings in the context of the employment sector, it is important to recognize that online postings can have very far-reaching consequences in other aspects of one's life. In a recent case in Texas, for example, a young woman had her baby taken away by state protective services due to the fact that the woman was found to be engaging in endangering conduct.[81] Among the evidence that the court considered in making its determination were photos from the woman's MySpace account, which had photos of her drinking alcohol, including captions that claimed she was drunk.[82] This case, along with others like it, emphasizes the necessity of discretion when using online social networking services.

The aforementioned cases are startling examples of the potential impacts of personal disclosures made online and, as such, demonstrate that people should be very cautious when contemplating the disclosure of information on the Internet. The lessons to be learned from these examples go far beyond the facts of the specific cases. As discussed earlier in this chapter, the ADA and other legislation protects you from certain intrusive medical questions from current and prospective employers. However, it is well established that many employers do use the Internet to conduct informal background checks on candidates.[83] Accordingly, if you are using social-networking sites and other online services in order to post private information about your health and any medical conditions that you may have, you may be providing your employer and prospective employers with access to information that these parties may not have otherwise been able to access and one never knows just how that information will impact you.

CONCLUSION

As this chapter has demonstrated, there are a number of health privacy issues that may arise in the workplace. While employers are not subject to HIPAA, they do have other privacy obligations. Employees, too, have their own role to play in protecting their privacy at work and should use caution and discretion in disclosing confidential medical information to your employer, co-workers or to the online world.

The next chapter, "Marketing Your Health," will examine how your medical information may be used for marketing, advertising, and promotions. HIPAA has always imposed fairly strict rules on the use of PHI for marketing purposes, and the HITECH Act further strengthened those limitations. Still, there are a number of ways in which information concerning your health may be used by a range of entities, sometimes without your knowledge and/or consent. For example, an area of growing concern—and increasing regulation—is the use of prescription data by data-mining companies to

6

Marketing Your Health

INTRODUCTION

There is a huge market for products and services geared toward health care and personal wellness. In 2008, more than $2.3 trillion was spent on health care.[1] In addition, while experiencing some recent declines, the pharmaceutical industry continues to be a source of great revenue, pulling in an estimated $291 billion in 2008.[2] Furthermore, factoring in the more loosely defined wellness industry (which may include things like gyms, supplements, massage, and other forms of personal care) would make these already high figures jump even higher.

Considering the current size and future growth potential of the health and wellness market, it is not too surprising that, medical and health information has become a valuable commodity for many marketers seeking to sell products and services. With knowledge about an individual's health status and medical conditions, a marketer can offer targeted sales messages to that person. For example, with the possession of a list of individuals who are receiving treatment for high blood pressure, a marketer will be well positioned to launch campaigns to market certain medications, nutritional supplements, exercise programs, and other treatments that may be of specific interest to those suffering from hypertension.

Companies that are able to collect details about individual health, medications, lifestyle, and behavior may be better positioned to market and sell various products and services, but at what cost to individual privacy? This chapter will examine the various marketing techniques that are being used in the health care industry and will explore the current legal environment impacting the ability of companies to market with medical information. It will also examine strategies for optimizing personal privacy protection.

HEALTH MARKETING AND THE LAW

HIPAA and the HITECH Act

The HIPAA Privacy Rule has long imposed fairly strict rules on the use of PHI for marketing purposes.[3] Under HIPAA, subject to certain limited exceptions that will be discussed further below, covered entities have been restricted from disclosing the PHI of an individual for marketing purposes unless that person grants authorization.

Understanding the definition of "marketing" has been key. Under the HIPAA Privacy Rule, "marketing" has had a two-part definition. First, "marketing" is "a communication about a product or service that encourages recipients of the communication to purchase or use the product or service." Generally, if the communication falls under this definition of "marketing," then the communication can occur only if the covered entity first obtains an individual's written authorization.[4] This general rule is subject to three exceptions[5] whereby the covered entity does not need the authorization of the individual if the communication is made: (i) to describe a health-related product or service that is provided by the covered entity making the communication; (ii) for the treatment of the individual; or (iii) for case management or care coordination for the individual, or to direct or recommend alternative treatments, therapies, health care providers, or settings of care to the individual.

Second, marketing also means "an arrangement between a covered entity and any other entity whereby the covered entity discloses protected health information to the other entity, in exchange for direct or indirect remuneration, for the other entity or its affiliate to make a communication about its own product or service that encourages recipients of the communication to purchase or use that product or service."[6] This part of the definition of marketing has no exceptions. Accordingly, a covered entity has been required to obtain the individual's prior authorization for any such disclosure of PHI. The purpose of this provision is to limit the sale of PHI.

There is a final distinction that should be noted as well. While the general rule has been that a covered entity must obtain an individual's authorization for any communication that meets the definition of marketing (unless an exception applies), a communication does not require an authorization, even if it is marketing, if it is (i) in the form of a face-to-face communication made by a covered entity to an individual; or (ii) a promotional gift of nominal value provided by the covered entity. As an example of a communication permitted by (i), a physician would not require your authorization to provide you with information about other products and services when you come in to see her for a consultation on a medical problem. As an example of a communication permitted by (ii), a hospital would not need patients' authorizations to provide new moms with samples of formula and other baby products of nominal value upon their discharge from the hospital.

The Health Information Technology for Economic and Clinical Health Act[7] (HITECH Act) has made significant changes to the rules governing the use of protected health information for marketing purposes. First, the HITECH Act has toughened the prohibition on selling PHI. Now, the HITECH Act will prohibit a covered entity or business associate from receiving direct or indirect payment in exchange for the PHI of any individual without the valid authorization from him or her.[8] However, the HITECH Act does provide six exceptions[9] permitting the sale of PHI when the sale is in exchange for (i) public health activities; (ii) research (but here, the price charged must reflect the costs of preparation and transmittal of the data); (iii) the treatment of an individual; (iv) health care operations related to the sale, transfer, merger, or consolidation of all or part of a covered entity and due diligence related to such activity; (v) providing an individual with a copy of his or her PHI; or (vi) other reasons determined necessary and appropriate by the Secretary of the Department of Health and Human Services (HHS). At the time of this writing, the implementation of these new requirements had not been finalized. However, HHS was required to promulgate regulations related to the sale of PHI and those regulations are expected to include important details that will dictate how providers are to implement the new requirements.[10]

The HITECH Act includes additional restrictions on permitted marketing communications. Under the changes introduced by the HITECH Act, a covered entity or business associate may not receive payment in exchange for the communication of PHI unless one of the following exceptions is met: (i) the communication describes only a drug or biologic that is currently being prescribed for the recipient of the communication, and payment received by the covered entity is reasonable; (ii) the communication is made by the covered entity with the authorization of the recipient of the communication; or (iii) the communication is made by a business associate that is consistent with the written contract between the business associate and the covered entity.[11] These requirements became effective on February 17, 2010.

State Law

When considering legal restrictions on marketing using health information, it is also important to consider state law. As you may recall, HIPAA basically sets a floor of protection but, for the most part, states can enact laws that provide stronger protection for health information. In this regard, California is particularly notable. Since 2005, California has had in place pretty strict legislation concerning the use of medical information for marketing purposes. California civil code §1798.91[12] prohibits companies from requesting an individual's medical information for marketing purposes without first obtaining consent from the individual and disclosing how the information will be used and disclosed. The requirement does not apply to businesses that are already required to obtain authorizations for the disclosure of medical information under the California Confidentiality of Medical Information Act. It also does not apply to some insurance and phone companies.

When a business wishes to orally obtain medical information from an individual, the law requires that it must orally disclose, in the same conversation as the request for the information, that the information is going to be used for marketing purposes and it must also obtain consent of the individual to whom the information pertains. The second requirement is particularly important since the law applies to obtaining medical information from an individual even when that information does not pertain to that person. The business will therefore have to still obtain consent from the individual whose information is to be used. If it is a written request for the information, however, the law requires a clear and conspicuous disclosure that the information will be used for marketing purposes and *written* consent from the individual to which the information pertains.

MARKETING USING AGGREGATED AND/OR DE-IDENTIFIED DATA

Although covered entities are generally prohibited from disclosing your PHI for marketing purposes without your authorization, the rules are different if your identity is removed. This is the concept of de-identification, and it is big business in health care marketing. "When health information does not identify an individual, and there is no reasonable basis to believe that it can be used to identify an individual, it is 'de-identified' and is not considered to be PHI."[13] Under HIPAA's Privacy Rule, "a [C]overed [E]ntity may use or disclose de-identified health information for any purpose without restriction."[14]

Given the broad rights that covered entities have been granted with respect to de-identified data, it is not very surprising that the HIPAA Privacy Rule has very specific rules concerning the requirements for de-identification of PHI. Under the HIPAA Privacy Rule, there are two methods for ensuring the de-identification of PHI. As the first option, a covered entity may determine that PHI has been de-identified if a person who is knowledgeable about and skilled in methods for de-identifying individually identifiable data:

(i) determines that the risk is very small that the information could be used, alone or in combination with other reasonably available information, by an anticipated recipient to identify an individual who is a subject of the information; and

(ii) documents the methods and results of the analysis that justify such determination.[15]

This essentially means that a person skilled in statistical analysis would need to be able to confirm that there is very little risk that the data in question could be used—alone or in combination with other reasonably available information—to identify the individual.

As a second option, a covered entity can effectively de-identify PHI by ensuring that the following identifiers of the individual or of relatives, employers, or household members of the individual are removed:

(A) Names;

(B) All geographic subdivisions smaller than a state, including street address, city, county, precinct, zip code, and their equivalent geocodes, except for the initial three digits of a zip code if, according to the current publicly available data from the Census:

   (1) The geographic unit formed by combining all zip codes with the same three initial digits contains more than 20,000 people; and

   (2) The initial three digits of a zip code for all such geographic units containing 20,000 or fewer people is changed to 000.

(C) All elements of dates (except year) for dates directly related to an individual, including birth date, admission date, discharge date, date of death; and all ages over 89 and all elements of dates (including year) indicative of such age, except that such ages and elements may be aggregated into a single category of age 90 or older;

(D) Telephone numbers;

(E) Fax numbers;

(F) E-mail addresses;

(G) Social Security numbers;

(H) Medical record numbers;

(I) Health plan beneficiary numbers;

(J) Account numbers;

(K) Certificate/license numbers;

(L) Vehicle identifiers and serial numbers, including license plate numbers;

(M) Device identifiers and serial numbers;

(N) Web universal resource locators (URLs);

(O) Internet protocol (IP) address numbers;

(P) Biometric identifiers, including fingerprints and voiceprints;

(Q) Full-face photographic images and any comparable images; and

(R) Any other unique identifying number, characteristic, or code.[16]

In addition to stripping out all of these identifiers, in order for the PHI at issue to be considered as de-identified, the covered entity could not have actual knowledge that the information could be used alone or in combination with other information to identify an individual who is a subject of the information.[17]

Despite the apparent clarity of the law, it is not always discernable when information has actually been de-identified. This is because it is possible to re-identify information even when no name is attached to it. Take an example with no severe consequence done as part of a privacy experiment by computer scientists at the University of Texas at Austin. The popular movie rental company Netflix held a competition to improve its recommendation software, and "anonymous" customers received a training data set containing the movie preferences of more than 480,000 customers who had been "de-identified." The computer scientists wanted to see if they could re-identify the unnamed movie fans. "By comparing the film preferences of some anonymous Netflix customers with personal profiles on http://www.imdb.com, the Internet movie database, the researchers said they easily re-identified some people because they had posted their e-mail addresses or other distinguishing information online."[18] Although the privacy concern is minimal for movie fans, it is easy to see a parallel to health information in an age that is increasingly becoming electronic. Currently, the clinical information systems market in the United States has sales of $8 to $10 billion a year with roughly 5 percent coming from data analysis.[19]

Since 2003, more than 45,000 complaints have been filed at the civil rights office in the Department of Health and Human Services by people who said their medical privacy was violated.[20] Many of these complaints come from individuals who have had some portion of their health information sold by many of the leading national pharmacies. "Companies that have been accused in lawsuits of buying and selling personal medical data include drugstore chains like Walgreens and data-mining companies like IMS Health and Verispan. CVS Caremark, which handles prescriptions for corporate clients, has also been accused of violating patients' privacy."[21] These companies all say that names of patients are removed or encrypted before data is sold, typically to drug manufacturers, but as the number of complaints suggests, there are often still breaches

For a concrete example, take the case of a California woman. More than 10 years ago, the woman tried unsuccessfully to become pregnant. She tried three different *in vitro* fertilization procedures and bought fertility drugs from her local pharmacy. Although her attempts were unsuccessful, the woman soon started receiving coupons and samples in the mail for products and services that would be needed by a family who had a baby at the time at which the woman was trying to have a baby. At first, she received coupons for diapers and baby formula, but over a period of 10 years, the advertisements continued, but changed to reflect a growing child. She received coupons for family photos and ideas for gifts for elementary school graduates. All were painful reminders of the child she was unable to have.[22]

The reason the woman received the information is because her pharmacy, like Walgreen's and CVS, has been able to accept payments from drug makers to mail advice and reminders to customers without obtaining permission. Currently, this practice is still legal as long as the information sent to consumers promotes only the drugs customers already buy.[23]

Quite recently, the utility of de-identification has come under further fire by researchers. In October 2009, a research study led by Dr. Khaled El Emam, the Canada Research Chair in Electronic Health Information at the CHEO Research Institute, revealed that purported de-identified information in hospital prescription records can be used quite easily to re-identify information believed to have been effectively de-identified.[24] And this is not the first time that concerns over the effectiveness of de-identification have been raised. In 2008, the National Institutes of Health (NIH) removed the DNA profiles of 60,000 patients from a public database because a study revealed that a new type of analysis could be used to confirm identities and that patients' genetic identities were not as anonymous as researchers previously believed them to be.[25]

This is surely not the last we will hear on the issue of de-identification. The HITECH Act required that HHS issue guidelines on how to de-identify PHI. To this end, in March 2010, the OCR put together a workshop to gather experts to exchange views on de-identification current practices, problems, and limitations.[26]

Prescription Data Mining

Marketing health information could not be the booming business it is without data miners. They are the companies that track prescriptions and then sell the information to drug manufacturers. It has been a large business for years. "Data miners say their research is valuable because gathering and analyzing information from thousands of people helps identify trends and provides indications of potentially dangerous side effects of drugs."[27] Data mining companies sell de-identified patient data to researchers or drug companies looking for patients to participate in clinical trials.[28] The prescription drug industry spends $30 billion a year in advertising; $7 billion a year is spent in direct advertising to physicians.[29]

Today, de-indentified health information makes up the majority of the work being done by data-mining companies such as IMS Health. In just the first half of 2009, IMS Health reported operating revenue of $1.05 billion.[30] By 2020, it is predicted that data-mining companies will be able to generate sales of up to $5 billion a year.[31]

The Issues

Most retail pharmacies store a large amount of prescription data in electronic databases. Typically, this data consists of the patient's name and contact information, the prescriber's name and contact information, as well as details about the prescribed medication (including type and brand of drug, dosage, and quantity).[32] Data-mining companies purchase stored prescription data from pharmacies and then aggregate, process, and sell the modified data to pharmaceutical companies.[33] Through a process termed "detailing," pharmaceutical sales representatives use the data to direct targeted marketing efforts toward specific physicians.[34] Detailing is said to occur when a representative from a pharmaceutical company communicates with a health care professional to provide information about pharmaceuticals and to promote particular pharmaceutical products.[35] Prescription data mining is viewed as a very effective process for marketers. With data from prescription histories, "marketers can see who's prescribing the competition's products and tailor pitches to convert them; who isn't prescribing much of anything and try to change that; and who are big prescribers and reward them, cultivating even more business."[36] There are a number of concerns about prescription data mining. Preeminent among them are privacy considerations. Sales of prescriber data take place without the consent, and generally without even the knowledge, of the prescribing physicians. The records are not to be identifiable to any particular individual. However, as noted in the prior section of this chapter, there are growing concerns about the effectiveness of current methods of de-identification. Patient privacy may be particularly vulnerable when records are sold from prescribing physicians in small communities with few physicians or few patients with particular diagnoses. The practice has also been criticized for having a negative impact on public health, based on the allegation that this kind of marketing based on prescriber data often involves biased and inaccurate information about health risks and encourages the prescription of new drugs that might be riskier to patients than already established treatments.[37] Opponents to the practice have also claimed that this type of marketing is a key factor in the continually rising costs of prescription drugs and the growth in use of expensive brand-name drugs.[38]

The practice of prescription data mining, while raising a number of significant privacy concerns, is not prohibited by HIPAA. While the HIPAA Privacy Rule restricts the ability of pharmacies to sell an individual's PHI for marketing purposes, HIPAA does not restrict a pharmacy from selling prescription data—identifiable to the prescribing physician (instead of the individual patient). Still, people may not want their prescription data sold—even when in aggregated, de-identified format. The practice may be even more objectionable to physicians who may not want their prescription records sold and who may not want to be subjected to targeted marketing based on the prescribing history. As a result of these concerns, a number of constituencies have been taking steps to attempt to limit the practice of prescription data mining.

The Law

New Hampshire was the first state to pass legislation to curb prescription mining. The measure, the New Hampshire Prescription Confidentiality Law,[39] was introduced by Representative Cindy Rosenwald, the wife of a cardiologist. The New Hampshire Medical Society supported the measure.[40] The New Hampshire law banned the use of prescription data linked to pre-scribers and patients for the purpose of targeting marketing to patients and doctors. It is important to note that the law did not prohibit the use of prescription data for marketing purposes. Rather, it merely required that companies only compile and use information regarding prescription drug sales in aggregated form so as to protect patients' individual prescription drug purchasing practices.

The New Hampshire Prescription Law was challenged by two data-mining companies on Constitutional grounds. The First Circuit Court, in *IMS Health v. Ayotte*, upheld the law, contending that the law did not violate the First Amendment because the law regulates conduct[41] (and not speech) and, further, that it did not violate the Commerce Clause because it affects only in-state transactions.[42] The case was then appealed to the U.S. Supreme Court, where the Court subsequently issued a release on June 29, 2009, declining to review the First Circuit's decision.[43]

In addition to New Hampshire's law, Maine and Vermont have similar laws on the books. Maine's law,[44] however, goes even farther than New Hampshire's law by "allow[ing] Maine doctors to opt out of participation in data mining, which would prevent a prescription drug information company from licensing, selling, or getting any value from transferring a doctor's pre-scribing information."[45]

Like the Vermont law, the Maine law also faced legal challenge. IMS Health Incorporated, Verispan, LLC, and Source Healthcare Analytics, Inc., three companies that collect identifying information about prescribing behaviors and analyze them for use in pharmaceutical marketing, challenged the law claiming that the restrictions violated the U.S. Constitution. However, on August 4, 2010, the U.S. Court of Appeals for the First Circuit upheld the Maine law, finding that the law did not violate the right to free speech of companies that collect identifying data about individual medical profession-als that prescribe drugs and aggregate the data for use in marketing pharma-ceutical products.[46]

As for Vermont's law,[47] the U.S. Supreme Court recently declined to review the case of *IMS Health v. Ayotte*.[48] When the Supreme Court declined to review the case, the Vermont law went into effect.[49] Meanwhile, at least nine other states, including New York and California, have proposals that are similar to the laws of the New England states.[50] With the Vermont and

Maine laws surviving their legal challenges, it would not be surprising if other jurisdictions enacted similar legislation in the near future.

PROTECTING YOURSELF AGAINST UNWANTED MARKETING

This section assumes that you will have an interest in limiting the use of your medical information for marketing purposes. For many readers, this will likely be the case. For others, however, the loss of some aspects of one's privacy may be perceived as an acceptable trade-off for the receipt of valuable, targeted marketing offers. Whatever one's view on this issue, arguably it is important that people are aware of companies' use of their information and have the opportunity to participate or decline to participate in such marketing. Below are some tips for protecting yourself from unwanted marketing involving your medical information.

Be wary of sharing health-related information with companies that are not covered entities: As discussed throughout this book, for the most part, HIPAA's privacy rules will apply only to covered entities and, to a certain extent, their business associates. If you share health information with entities that are not subject to HIPAA, don't expect that they will protect your information in a manner that complies with HIPAA. You should be careful not only about express disclosures, such as information you may disclose when completing health surveys at spas and health clubs, for example, but also about information that you may disclose through your actions. For instance, you may wish to be cautious when using discount shopping cards. Those cards offer insight into your purchasing habits and, depending upon what you buy, may reveal information about a medical condition you may have. Depending upon applicable state law, and, unless the shop with which you have taken out the discount card has agreed otherwise, the store may be free to use your information for marketing purposes as it sees fit.

Read authorizations carefully and refused to sign authorizations you do not understand: Authorizations can be used in order to authorize covered entities to use and share your PHI in a number of ways, including for marketing purposes. Be sure that you read and understand an authorization before executing it and avoid signing any blanket authorizations.

Be careful what you disclose online: Once you disclose information online, it will be next to impossible to pull it back. You will also lose control over who can access and use the information and for what purposes. Exercise caution when disclosing information on public forums even when doing so on what you believe to be an anonymous basis.

Remove your name from direct-marketing lists: Where possible, opt out of the sharing of your personal information by entities with which you do business. Remove yourself from mailing lists.[51]

CONCLUSION

Your medical information is extremely valuable to a lot of different constituencies. There are laws in place that put some limitations on the ability of various entities to use your information for marketing purposes. However, even with these laws in place, a very significant amount of marketing continues to occur. For some, these marketing practices may be viewed as beneficial as they can provide access to products and services that are valued. However, often people do not even know that their information is being used for various marketing-related activities, nor do they have an option to determine whether or not they approve of such use.

Chapter 7 will examine privacy issues related to special health conditions, such as substance abuse, mental illness, and sexually transmitted diseases. While all health information may be viewed as sensitive, information regarding the types of illnesses discussed in Chapter 7 is among the most sensitive information. Unauthorized disclosures of PHI concerning the types of illnesses discussed in the next chapter can have significant consequences for the individual concerned. It is thus not too surprising that there are stronger laws in place to protect this most sensitive information.

7

The Special Cases of Mental Health, Addiction, Socially Stigmatizing Diseases, and Other Intensely Private Health Matters

INTRODUCTION

This chapter focuses on conditions that may have special privacy considerations, such as mental health disorders, addiction problems, socially stigmatizing diseases, and reproductive issues. While protecting the privacy of all medical information is important, privacy is particularly significant insofar as these kinds of conditions are concerned. There are a number of potential implications for disclosures of details regarding mental health disorders, substance abuse problems, and sexually transmitted diseases (STDs), including possible employment discrimination, insurance discrimination, social stigmatization, the destruction of familial and/or social relationships, and even, with respect to data regarding substance abuse, for instance, criminal penalties.

The fear of possibly experiencing such consequences may result in ill people failing to seek care when needed. The avoidance of proper treatment for these kinds of ailments can have negative repercussions not only for the individual, but also for his or her community and society at large. Thus, the need to protect the privacy and security of this kind of information goes far beyond a mere desire to respect the privacy of the individual; it actually is an issue of safety and proper patient care.

In order to give proper diagnoses and treatments, health care professionals must have an in-depth knowledge about a patient's medical history, including any mental health conditions and/or any problems with substance abuse. However, patient information regarding these conditions is among the most sensitive types of information. Achieving the appropriate balance between providing proper health care quality and optimum patient safety on the one hand,

and ensuring patient confidentiality on the other hand, has been a challenge for health care providers and policymakers alike for some time now and will likely continue to be so. The tension between these two important goals is particularly evident when dealing with patient information of individuals who are seeking treatment for mental health disorders and/or substance abuse problems.

Another area of tension is found between the need to protect individual privacy and the need to protect the public health and other individuals. This tension is evident in connection with many of the illnesses discussed in this chapter. Consider, for instance, an individual who is under treatment for a substance abuse problem. While there are important reasons for protecting the person's privacy, such interests may be at odds with the need to protect the public if, for example, the individual is in a position where his or her substance abuse problem can result in harm to the public, such as, for example, if they are an airline pilot, school bus driver, or surgeon. The same tension exists with STDs. While those who are afflicted with these diseases certainly have privacy interests to protect, these interests are sometimes overridden by the need to protect the public from further transmission of these diseases.

Against this complicated background, this chapter explores the key federal and state protections that are in place to protect these various kinds of sensitive information. By exploring some key cases, it will also show the kinds of remedies that may be available to those who suffer a violation of their privacy in sensitive health information.

LEGAL PROTECTIONS FOR SENSITIVE HEALTH INFORMATION

Overview

One expert has described the law governing the confidentiality of health care information as a "crazy quilt of federal and state constitutional, statutory, regulatory, and case law" that "erodes personal privacy and forms a serious barrier to administrative simplification."[1] This comment, made prior to the enactment of the Health Insurance Portability and Accountability Act (HIPAA), remains largely applicable with respect to the sensitive health information that is the focus of this chapter.

Given the risks associated with access to sensitive health information, it is little wonder that many state laws, and some federal ones, afford a relatively higher degree of protection for some specialized categories of protected health information (PHI), such as data about one's HIV status, STD history, mental health treatment, and/or substance abuse problems, than the protections that are available under HIPAA for more general classes of PHI. By and large, legal protections for these sensitive classes of information were in place prior to HIPAA. Recall that HIPAA is a relatively recent creation, being enacted in 1996. However, many laws to protect the sensitive information discussed in this chapter were in place well in advance of HIPAA. For example, federal laws to protect the confidentiality of substance abuse records have been in place since the 1970s, and states began to enact legislation to protect the privacy of individuals' HIV status in the late 1980s and early 1990s.

The Problem of Consent

Many of the laws that provide enhanced protection for information related to potentially socially stigmatizing disorders require the individual's written consent or permission prior to any disclosure of certain sensitive health information. While requiring patient consent adds another layer of protection, these laws also raise numerous legal and practical issues. At a most basic level, people suffering from some of these ailments may not be in the best position to determine whether or not to consent to a particular use or disclosure of their information. For example, an individual suffering from an untreated mental illness, or someone who is actively abusing drugs or alcohol, may not fully understand the terms of a consent form and the implications of agreeing to its terms. From a practical perspective, there may also be questions about the content and format of the consent form that is used with patients. The consent form must be constructed and presented to ensure that the vulnerable patient understands and agrees to the proposed disclosure of information. Key issues likely to arise in connection with the drafting of the consent form include the degree of specificity; the type and quality of information that should be used in obtaining a patient's consent; the disclosure of his or her health information to other providers; and how long a written permission should be considered effective before the patient must sign it again.

Federal Law

As noted earlier in the book, HIPAA creates a federal "floor" of privacy protections; it establishes minimum protections for PHI while allowing states to enact more stringent laws. It is also important to note that HIPAA does not displace other federal laws; separate and more protective federal privacy standards applicable to certain PHI must be considered in tandem with HIPAA. Given this reality, it can be difficult for individuals to understand the full scope and limitations of privacy protections.

With very limited exceptions, the HIPAA Privacy Rule does not distinguish between types of data that are included within the definition of PHI.[2] It does, however, recognize that some existing federal and state privacy and confidentiality laws accord greater protection for certain types of health information and leaves these laws undisturbed.

In general, the HIPAA Privacy Rule permits a covered entity to use and disclose PHI for certain core purposes—such as treatment, payment, and health care operations—without requiring an individual's prior written consent. The rule permits a covered entity to share patient information with another treating professional. For most purposes, including payment and health care operations, the HIPAA Privacy Rule limits covered entities' uses, disclosures, and requests of PHI from other covered entities to the minimum amount necessary to accomplish the intended purpose of the use or disclosure; this is known as the "minimum necessary" rule.[3] However, this rule does not apply to requests for, or disclosures of, PHI for treatment purposes.[4] In other words, HIPAA allows providers to share any PHI in the patient's medical record for treatment purposes.

No written authorization is needed when PHI is being provided to the individual who is the subject of the information. In fact, disclosure to the person himself or herself is one of only two required disclosures (the other is to the Secretary of the Department of Health and Human Services for purposes of auditing the covered entity for compliance). Similarly, if the individual is present and has an opportunity to either agree or object in the case of disclosures to family members or others involved in their care, no written authorization is needed.[5]

The HIPAA Privacy Rule allows covered entities flexibility to maintain their own framework for the use or disclosure of PHI by establishing a series of categories for permissive disclosures. This structure facilitates the ability of health care professionals to continue many of their existing privacy practices, thus allowing them to develop their own approach to health information privacy in key care areas as long as their policies and practices are explained in writing to their patients in advance.

Covered entities may also use and disclose protected health information without an individual's written permission for a variety of national priority purposes, including health care oversight, public health, research, law enforcement, and when other laws require disclosure.[6] Outside of treatment, payment, and health care operations, or the permissive exceptions noted above, the HIPAA Privacy Rule requires that entities obtain written permission from patients prior to the use or disclosure of PHI. These "authorizations" must meet specific content and format requirements. Additionally, psychotherapy notes are covered by a special authorization rule.

Recall from Chapter 2 that, while HIPAA provides patients with broad rights of access to medical information, patients *do not* have the right to access a provider's psychotherapy notes. These notes, taken by a mental health professional during a conversation with a patient, are kept separate from the patient's medical and billing records. The HIPAA Privacy Rule also does not permit the provider to make most disclosures of psychotherapy notes about you without your authorization.

Under HIPAA, authorizations must be written in plain language and contain:

- A specific and meaningful description of the information to be disclosed or used;
- The name or specific identification of the person(s) authorized to disclose the information;
- The name or specific identification of the person(s) to whom the information can be disclosed;
- A description of each purpose of the requested use or disclosure;
- An expiration date or event;
- The signature of the individual and date; and
- A few required statements to place the individual on notice of his/her rights, including the right to revoke consent.[7]

In the case of disclosures of PHI to a business associate, a covered entity must enter into an agreement with the business associate that includes assurances that the business associate will appropriately safeguard PHI.

Confidentiality of Alcohol and Drug Abuse Records under Federal Law

Since the early 1970s, patient records for alcohol and drug abuse treatment have been entitled to special provider/patient confidentiality protections under federal law.[8] These laws have important implications for the electronic exchange of health information. The federal Confidentiality of Alcohol and Drug Abuse Patient Records law, reflecting Congressional concern about the potential negative impacts of seeking alcohol and drug treatment, creates a virtual shield against the disclosure of information related to these types of conditions and treatment. Its implementing regulations[9] have become such a staple of the legal landscape that they are known simply as Part 2 of the broader body of federal substance use regulations of which they are a part.

With certain conditions and exceptions, Part 2 strictly prohibits the disclosure of drug and alcohol use records maintained in connection with the performance of any federally assisted alcohol and/or drug program.

To understand the significance of the prohibitions of the law, it is necessary to understand the key definitions. First, note that federal assistance is defined very broadly, and includes being (1) conducted in whole or in part by any U.S. department or agency; (2) licensed, certified, registered, or otherwise authorized by any U.S. department or agency (including being certified with provider status under the Medicare program, being authorized to conduct methadone maintenance treatment, or being registered to dispense controlled substances); (3) supported by funds provided by any U.S. department or agency, including as a recipient of federal financial assistance in any form (not limited to the provision of substance abuse or alcohol treatment), con-ducted by a state or local government that receives federal funds that could be used for alcohol or drug abuse treatment, or is assisted by the IRS through the allowance of contributions as tax deductions.[10]

Disclosure means a "communication of patient identifying information, the affirmative verification of another person's communication of patient identifying information, or the communication of any information from the record of a patient who has been identified."[11] Patient-identifying informa-tion includes names, addresses, Social Security numbers, fingerprints, pho-tographs, or "similar information by which the identity of a patient can be determined with reasonable accuracy and speed either directly or by reference to other publicly available information."[12] Criminal penalties for violations include a fine of not more than $500 for first offenses and not more than $5,000 for each subsequent offense.[13]

Part 2 sweeps broadly in defining both patients and programs. Its provi-sions are stringent, prohibiting disclosure of any information[14] that could either directly or indirectly identify an individual as an alcohol or substance abuse patient.[15]

Part 2 applies to "programs," which are defined as individuals or enti-ties (other than general medical facilities) or identified units within general medical facilities that hold themselves out as providing and that actually do provide alcohol or drug abuse diagnosis, treatment, or referral for treatment; or medical personnel or other staff in a general medical care facility whose primary function is the provision of alcohol or drug abuse diagnosis, treat-ment, or referral for treatment and who are identified as such providers.[16]

"Patient" is also defined broadly by Part 2 to include any individual who has applied for or been given a diagnosis or treatment for alcohol or drug abuse at a federally assisted program and includes any person who, after an arrest on a criminal charge, is identified as an alcohol or drug abuser in order to determine eligibility to participate in a program.[17]

Importantly, all permissible disclosures under Part 2 are limited to "infor-mation that is necessary to carry out the purpose of the disclosure."[18] While Part 2 prohibits the use of covered information to form the basis of a criminal charge,[19] the law requires disclosure in response to a subpoena issued as part of an ongoing court procedure pursuant to an authorizing court order.[20]

Part 2's restrictions on disclosure allow certain exceptions, the most perti-nent of which for our purposes are (1) communications within a program or between a program and an entity having direct administrative control over that program; and (2) the granting of tax-exempt status to the program.[21] There are special exceptions for information on alcohol and drug abuse patients main-tained in connection with the Department of Veterans Affairs and other limits for information obtained by the Armed Forces.[22]

Outside of the exceptions just discussed, nearly all disclosures under Part 2 require specific patient consent, and its content and format must meet the federal standards described below. In contrast, the HIPAA Privacy Rule does not require any consent to disclose PHI for treatment, payment, or health care operation purposes. If a provider elects to obtain such consent, he or she is permitted under HIPAA to use a general consent form. Thus, Part 2's "specific consent" format sets a far higher bar than HIPAA with respect to consent requirements.

The required elements of a Part 2 consent form are:

1) The name of the patient;
2) The purpose of the disclosure;
3) How much and what kind of information is to be disclosed;
4) The signature of the patient (or if a minor, incompetent, or deceased, then the signature of a person authorized to give consent);
5) The date the consent is signed;
6) A statement that the consent is subject to revocation at any time except to the extent that the discloser has acted in reliance;
7) The date, event, or condition upon which the consent will expire, if not revoked before; and
8) A statement that the information being disclosed may not be re-disclosed without the individual's consent.[23]

As with HIPAA, Part 2 sets a federal privacy "floor," preempting state laws that are less protective while allowing state laws that are more stringent to apply.[24] As a result, if you are concerned about the type of information that may be subject to the protections of Part 2, it would be wise to consult not only the provisions of Part 2, but also the provisions of any applicable state laws that may offer greater protections.

The Role of the Family Educational Rights and Privacy Act of 1974

The Family Educational Rights and Privacy Act of 1974[25] (FERPA) protects the privacy of student education records, serving two main functions:

1. To create a right of access to student records for parents and students; and
2. To protect the privacy of those records by preventing unauthorized access by third parties.

FERPA prohibits the release of education records without parental consent, or, in the case of students age 18 or older or attending college, without the consent of the student.[26] FERPA applies to all public or private educational agencies at the elementary, secondary, and higher education level that receive federal education funding. "Protected records" is defined broadly under

FERPA and can include information related to the treatment of a student for substance abuse or mental health conditions. Under FERPA, student records are records, files, documents, and other materials that contain information directly related to a student and are maintained by an educational agency or institution or by a person acting for such an agency or institution.[27] Records of both current and former students are covered. For a record to be protected by FERPA, it must contain personally identifiable information about a student. FERPA does provide for a set of circumstances in which disclosures without consent are allowed. However, parental or (where appropriate) student consent is required to release educational records involving medical treatment.

Records covered by FERPA are not subject to HIPAA because HIPAA's definition of PHI specifically excludes FERPA records.[28] This means that unlike Part 2, HIPAA and FERPA do not overlap. Thus, FERPA adds an extra layer to federal health information law and the policy protections regarding confidentiality of records.

Medicaid Privacy Statute

The Medicaid privacy statute is a precursor to HIPAA. While its provisions bear a striking resemblance to the basic HIPAA rule, HHS has not issued a formal interpretation aligning Medicaid privacy standards squarely with the HIPAA Privacy Rule. This lack of action by HHS has created a fair amount of confusion.

Federal Medicaid law requires state plans for medical assistance to provide safeguards that restrict the use and disclosure of patient information to purposes directly connected with administration of the plan, defined as establishing eligibility, determining the amount of medical assistance, providing services for recipients, and conducting or assisting investigations, prosecutions, or legal proceedings related to the administration of the plan.[29]

Additionally, the implementing regulations require agencies to establish criteria for safeguarding specific information about applicants and recipients, including at least the following information:

- Names;
- Addresses;
- Medical services provided;
- Social and economic conditions and circumstances;
- Agency evaluations of personal information;
- Medical data, including diagnosis and history of disease or disability;
- Information received for verifying income eligibility and amount of medical assistance payments; and
- Information received in connection with the identification of legally liable third-party resources.

The regulations also require agencies to have criteria specifying conditions for the release and use of information about applicants and recipients. Access to this information is restricted to individuals who are subject to standards of confidentiality comparable to those of the agency. With certain exceptions, the regulations also require permission from a family member or individual, wherever possible, before an agency can respond to an information request from an outside source. Additionally, agencies must have data exchange agreements (similar to HIPAA business associate agreements) in order to exchange data with other agencies.

Thus, as with HIPAA, the Medicaid statute outlines a basic floor of privacy and for the use of formal protocols to guide data disclosures. Unlike HIPAA, however, Medicaid does not appear to address patient consent for disclosure in the context of treatment, payment, and health care operations as a general rule. Instead, it appears, like FERPA and Part 2, to rely on the more traditional approach of requiring specific patient consent for disclosures of personally identifiable information.

State Privacy Laws Governing Sensitive Health Issues

Overview

States also play an important role in protecting the privacy of sensitive medical data. Many states have enacted legislation to protect data concerning particularly sensitive medical issues, such as information pertaining to HIV, STDs, substance use, and mental health issues. As mentioned above, it is important to recall that HIPAA merely sets a minimum standard for information protection. There is nothing stopping states from imposing stricter protections; HIPAA only preempts state laws that provide less protection. As such, in many states, the proscribed protection for information concerning HIV, STDs, and substance abuse is more stringent than the requirements set out in the HIPAA Privacy Rule.

Just as HIPAA requires specific patient consent for disclosures of information related to HIV, STDs, and substance abuse, the most common exception to confidentiality in state law is when the person who is or has been in treatment consents to a waiver of confidentiality. Most state laws differ from the federal provisions, however, in that the form the consent must take to be valid is not explicitly stated.[30]

Also like HIPAA, there are many states with provisions in their mental health confidentiality laws that allow the disclosure of confidential information when it is necessary to obtain reimbursement or other financial assistance for the person in treatment. There are, however, some exceptions. For example, New Jersey restricts disclosure of information from licensed psychologists to third-party payers. The statute permits disclosure only if the patient consents, and if disclosure is limited to (1) administrative information; (2) diagnostic information; (3) the legal status of the patient; (4) the reason for continuing psychological services; (5) assessment of the patient's current level of functioning and level of distress; and (6) a prognosis, limited to the minimal time treatment might continue.[31]

New York serves as a leading example of how state laws can provide enhanced protections over what is provided under the HIPAA Privacy Rule. New York's Mental Hygiene Law, which includes provisions addressing the rights of patients,[32] is similar in many respects to HIPAA. There are, however, some subtle differences, and the New York law includes parts that are stricter than HIPAA. For example, HIPAA permits PHI to be released without patient consent in the course of any judicial or administrative proceeding if the covered entity has made reasonable efforts to give the patient notice of the request or if the covered entity is assured that reasonable efforts have been made to secure a qualified protective order. But New York permits disclosure only after a "finding that the interests of justice significantly outweigh the need for confidentiality."[33]

Regarding the release of patient information, HIPAA allows a covered entity "to use/disclose PHI to the patient (including a patient's personal representative, i.e., someone authorized to act on patient's behalf to make health care decisions)."[34] New York law, however, permits this information to be disclosed only to those "who have a demonstrable need for such information provided such disclosure will not reasonably be expected to be detrimental to the patient or others."[35]

State Laws Concerning Information about HIV/AIDS

Overview

Many states began to focus on the privacy of information concerning HIV/AIDS in the late 1980s and 1990s. As people became more aware about AIDS, public fear of the disorder grew. As a result, individuals who were suffering from AIDS or were HIV-positive became subject to discrimination. At the same time, public health officials became concerned that, due to the discrimination that HIV-positive people often suffered, they would be reluctant to get tested if the privacy of their information could not be assured.[36] As a result, many state lawmakers began to identify a need to protect the privacy of information concerning individuals' HIV status, a need that was summed up very well by the New Jersey Supreme Court in a 1991 opinion.

Individuals infected with HIV are concerned with maintaining the confidentiality of their health status. HIV infection is associated with sexual practice and drug use, universally regarded as personal and sensitive activities. In addition, the majority of people infected with HIV in the United States are members of groups that are traditionally disfavored. Even before the AIDS epidemic, gays and intravenous drug users were subject to persistent prejudice and discrimination. AIDS brings with it a special stigma. Attitude surveys show that even though most Americans understand the modes through which HIV is spread, a significant minority still would exclude those who are HIV-positive from schools, public accommodations, and the workplace. Unauthorized disclosure of a person's serologic status can lead to social opprobrium among family and friends, as well as loss of employment, housing, and insurance.[37]

Today, the vast majority of states have laws that protect the privacy of data concerning an individual's HIV status. In addition, many states (including Arizona, California, Delaware, Hawaii, Illinois, Maine, Montana, New Hampshire, New York, North Dakota, Ohio, Oklahoma, Pennsylvania, Vermont, Virginia, West Virginia, and Wisconsin) allow for civil liability for actual damages, costs, and attorneys' fees.[38] In some states (including Arizona, Colorado, Florida, Georgia, Idaho, Iowa, Kansas, Montana, North Carolina, South Dakota, and Utah), violators of the restrictions on the disclosure of HIV information may be charged with misdemeanors and can be subject to fines and imprisonment.[39]

New York is an example of a state that provides strong protections to the privacy of data regarding HIV and AIDS. For one, under New York state law, HIV testing generally requires the informed written consent of the testing subject.[40] The consent form must explain the protections afforded under the law to HIV-related information, including the circumstances under which, and the persons to whom, disclosure of information may be required, authorized, or permitted by law.[41]

New York law also places tight controls on the disclosure of HIV-related information. A person who obtains confidential HIV-related information in the course of providing health or social services, or pursuant to a release, cannot disclose such information except, as specified in the statute, to the protected individual or his representative; any person to whom disclosure is authorized pursuant to a release; an agent or employee of a health facility or health care provider under certain circumstances; a health care provider or facility when the information is necessary to care for the individual, the individual's child, or one of the individual's contacts; a federal, state, county, or local health officer when such disclosure is mandated by federal or state law; third-party reimbursers; insurance institutions under certain circumstances; and others.[42] Those who disclose confidential HIV-related information in violation of the law are subject to a maximum civil penalty of $5,000 per occurrence.[43] Those who willfully commit violations are guilty of misdemeanors and subject to additional penalties.

Reporting Requirements

While the majority of states do provide strong protections for the privacy of information concerning HIV/AIDS, in many states, there are also some reporting requirements that can invade the privacy of afflicted individuals. One of the most notable is a South Carolina law that requires the state Department of Health and Environmental Control (DHEC) to report the identities of HIV-positive public school students to school officials.[44] Reporting requirements like this are very concerning, as available data demonstrates that HIV-positive children report stigmatization and harassment when people at their school learn of their status.[45] As a result, these reporting requirements may not only infringe upon the health privacy rights of individuals and cause them to suffer harassment and discrimination, but they may also have a chilling effect on the willingness of others to undergo HIV testing. This is startling when one considers the fact that 25 percent of HIV-positive people are unaware of their status.[46] Our laws should be designed to promote and encourage testing, not discourage it by making people fearful of what will occur once they receive their results.

State Laws Concerning Mental Health Issues

As was the case with HIV data, state laws are also very protective with respect to information concerning mental health disorders. There is a clear rationale for these provisions. Despite a greater acceptance of the notion that mental health disorders should be treated like physical ailments and should not be the subject of shame, embarrassment, or disdain, individuals seeking and obtaining mental health services are still often stigmatized.[47] Accordingly, if as a matter of public policy, we wish to ensure that those who need mental health services are not discouraged from seeking help due to the prospects of stigma, it will be essential to ensure that their privacy will be protected.

The vast majority of states provide statutory protections for records concerning mental health treatment. However, fewer than half of the states provide for civil or criminal remedies of the unauthorized disclosure of mental health treatment records. In a small number of states (including the District of Columbia, Colorado, Hawaii, Illinois, Iowa, Kansas, Kentucky, Nebraska, South Carolina, Utah, and Wyoming), individuals who violate state laws concerning the disclosure of mental health records can be charged with a misdemeanor and may be subject to fines and/or imprisonment.

By means of example, consider legislation in place in Utah. Utah law provides that a psychologist, licensed substance abuse counselor, or mental health therapist may not disclose any confidential communication with a client or patient without that patient's or his authorized agent's express consent (a parent or guardian if the patient is a minor).[48] Disclosure of this protected information without the prior authorization of the patient is permitted in a limited number of circumstances, such as when necessary to respond to state reporting requirements, when the disclosure is made as part of an administrative, civil, or criminal proceeding, and when disclosure of information is made under a generally recognized professional or ethical standard that authorizes or requires disclosure.[49]

State Laws Concerning STD Information

In addition to the laws that target HIV/AIDS more specifically, a number of jurisdictions have enacted laws to protect the privacy of information concerning other STDs. The majority of states have laws that require that information concerning STDs be protected as confidential, while also imposing reporting requirements to state health officials. However, only a minority of states provide civil or criminal remedies for violations of the non-disclosure requirements.

Consider the law of Pennsylvania on this issue. Pennsylvania law requires that physicians report those who have or who are suspected of having a communicable disease to the local board or department of health.[50] Similar reporting obligations apply to clinical laboratories, health care practitioners, health care facilities, orphanages, childcare group settings, and institutions maintaining dormitories and living rooms.[51] Health authorities are prohibited from disclosing these reports to anyone outside the department except when necessary to control or prevent communicable disease.[52] In addition, the law authorizes researchers to use the reports, subject to strict supervision, to ensure that their use is limited to the specific research purposes.[53] Individuals who violate the nondisclosure rules can be subject to fines and, when the fine is unpaid, imprisonment.[54]

NOTABLE CASE LAW

Breaches and/or invasions of privacy involving the kind of information discussed in this chapter may be particularly damaging and may open the door for possible lawsuits. As discussed, HIPAA does not allow for a private right of action, meaning that individuals who have suffered an invasion of privacy due to a covered entity's violation of HIPAA will not be able to sue for damages suffered under HIPAA. However, as will be shown through the following case examples, those who have suffered certain privacy violations of their medical information may find that they can pursue claims under state law.

Given the particular sensitivity surrounding information about one's HIV status, it is not surprising—but it is very unfortunate—that there have been a number of cases concerning claims of privacy violations for the unauthorized disclosure of information about an individual's HIV status. One notable case was decided in the Ninth Circuit, where the court reversed a lower court's ruling for summary judgment, finding that a plaintiff seeking recovery under the Privacy Act of 1974[55] could seek damages for humiliation, mental anguish, and emotional distress caused by the unauthorized disclosure of his medical information by government agencies. The underlying case concerned a plaintiff who was diagnosed as being HIV-positive. Subsequent to this diagnosis, he was subject to a criminal investigation wherein the validity of his pilot's license was called into question. The plaintiff claimed that during the course of this investigation, various government agencies exchanged information about his HIV status, thereby violating the federal Privacy Act.

In defending the plaintiff's suit, the government contended that the plaintiff suffered no "actual damages" under the Privacy Act because he only claimed non-pecuniary injuries. Although the lower court found a violation of the federal Privacy Act, it agreed with government's contention that the plaintiff had not suffered any actual harm. In making its finding, the lower court primarily relied on the fact that it believed there was ambiguity as to whether emotional distress qualified as "actual damages" under the Privacy Act. As such, in order to award damages against the government, the court must find that the government expressly waived sovereign immunity, which it did not under the Privacy Act.[56] However, on appeal, the Ninth Circuit concluded that the Privacy Act does allow for the recovery of damages for non-pecuniary injuries, such as the humiliation, mental anguish, and emotional distress allegedly suffered by the plaintiff. This is a significant ruling as it affirms an avenue of recourse for individuals who may experience the unauthorized use and/or disclosure of their sensitive medical information (such as HIV status) by governmental agencies who are subject to the federal Privacy Act.

Lawsuits for violations involving information about one's HIV status are not new. In some jurisdictions, cases were brought even before legislation was in place to protect the confidentiality of HIV information. Consider, for instance, one 1991 case from New Jersey.[57] This case involved an otolaryngologist who, after being ill for several weeks, was admitted to a local hospital where he held staff privileges. Testing at the hospital revealed that he was HIV-positive, a finding that neither he nor his treating physician had previously suspected. After being discharged from the hospital, the patient returned home to a series of phone calls from physicians, none of whom were involved in his care, but all of whom had apparent knowledge of his condition. News of the otolaryngologist's condition soon spread to the larger community, and he became socially ostracized and also experienced a significant contraction in his medical practice.

The otolaryngologist sued the medical center and his treating physician for breaching his confidentiality. Although the plaintiff was not able to identify the precise source of the unauthorized disclosure of information regarding his HIV status, he alleged that the widespread dissemination of information about his health status showed that the defendants had failed to take reasonable measures to prevent unauthorized access to his test results.

In finding the medical center responsible for the breach of confidentiality, the court stated:

The confidentiality breached in the present case in simply grist for a gossip mill with little concern from the impact of the disclosure on the patient. While one can legitimately question the good judgment of a practicing physician choosing to undergo HIV testing or a bronchoscopy procedure at the same hospital where he practices, this apparent error in judgment does not relieve the medical center of its underlying obligation—to protect its patients against the dissemination of confidential information. It makes little difference to identify those who "spread the news." The information was too easily available, too titillating to disregard. All that was required was a glance at a chart, and the written words became whispers and the whispers became roars. And common sense told all that this would happen.[58]

Cases involving the unauthorized disclosure of data concerning HIV status continue in the current era. Another interesting case arose in 2004, when the Social Security Administration (SSA) agreed to pay a woman $65,000 for revealing her HIV-positive status.[59] In addition to the financial settlement, the SSA also agreed to prevent further dissemination of the woman's HIV status to unauthorized parties.[60] The underlying facts of this case are somewhat similar to those in the New Jersey case discussed above, in the sense that a rumor mill helped to spread information about an individual's HIV status. In this case, the plaintiff filed for disability benefits after she was unable to work due to depression and AIDS. In connection with her application for benefits, she was required to participate in an application interview with an SSA representative. The representative asked the plaintiff for information about her health history and her personal life. After the interview, the SSA representative told a mutual friend that the plaintiff had AIDS. Soon thereafter, news of the plaintiff's medical condition spread throughout their social circle.

The plaintiff brought a lawsuit, claiming that the SSA and the SSA employee who revealed the information about the plaintiff's health violated the Privacy Act and the plaintiff's constitutional right to privacy. She sought damages for the emotional harm she suffered, as well as an order prohibiting the SSA from further disclosing her health information.

Although this chapter has not focused upon information concerning reproductive issues, information about these kinds of matters is also particularly sensitive and its exposure can be quite harmful. As such, it is appropriate to briefly touch on the subject here. In 2007, the Appellate Division of the New York Supreme Court upheld a jury award of punitive damages for an unintentional privacy breach. In the case of *Randi A. J. v. Long Island Surgi-Center*,[61] the court ruled, in a 3–2 decision, that punitive damages may be awarded for a grossly negligent breach of confidential medical information—even if the breach was the result of negligence and was not intentional or malicious.[62] The court upheld the jury's award of $365,000 ($65,000 in compensatory emotional distress damages and $300,000 in punitive damages) despite acknowledging that the defendant was acting in good faith and without malice or intent to violate the plaintiff's privacy rights. According to the court's decision, a plaintiff does not have to prove malice or bad faith in order to be awarded punitive damages.[63]

The case involved a 20-year-old woman who underwent an abortion at the defendant surgery center.[64] When filling out a preoperative questionnaire, the plaintiff included her home telephone number, but then crossed it out. Because she lived with her parents and did not want them to know of the procedure (her parents were opposed to abortion), she gave specific instructions to only call her cell phone. But administrative personnel at the surgery center generated patient file labels that included her home number, and a nurse later made a call to that number to follow up on lab tests. Despite realizing that she was speaking with the patient's mother, the nurse proceeded to discuss the patient's condition in a manner that made apparent the fact that the plaintiff had undergone an abortion.[65]

The court found that although the defendant did not act in bad faith, the actions of the center and its personnel rose to the level of recklessness and gross negligence, specifically pointing out that the center had no written policy for protecting the patient's right to privacy and confidentiality.[66]

These cases show how, notwithstanding the lack of a private right of action for privacy violations under HIPAA, those who suffer losses as a result of breaches of privacy concerning their sensitive medical information may have legal recourse under applicable state laws.

CONCLUSION

While many individuals are concerned about the privacy of their health information, those suffering from mental health ailments, STDs, and/or substance abuse problems may have particularly pressing reasons to wish that their medical information remains private and secure. As this chapter has demonstrated, in addition to HIPAA, other federal and state laws play a role in the protection of health information concerning these kinds of ailments. These enhanced protections are necessary because without sufficient assurances of privacy and data security, individuals suffering from these problems may be reluctant to seek treatment and care.

Chapter 8 will introduce international perspectives on health privacy. As the nation begins to implement sweeping reforms to our health care system and continues to contemplate the possibility of other changes, it is important to keep analyzing advantages and disadvantages of other systems. This chapter will explore a number of key jurisdictions around the world and discuss how they seek to ensure the protection of individual health privacy rights.

8

International Perspectives on Health Privacy

INTRODUCTION

The United States has a fairly comprehensive and strong legislative regime in place to ensure the privacy and security of individual medical information. The American culture is not the only one that places a high value on privacy rights. In fact, many countries have stronger and/or more comprehensive privacy laws than in the United States. Additionally, many of the countries with strong privacy laws also have longer histories of protecting privacy. As we continue to evaluate the efficacy and the shortcomings of the American system, it is useful to consider how medical privacy is protected in other countries.

While the privacy laws under investigation in this chapter are generally more protective than those in place in the United States, these other systems are not flawless. In fact, in each of the jurisdictions investigated in this chapter, there have been a number of highly publicized data breaches involving medical information.[1] Additionally, in many of the jurisdictions, there continues to be contentious debates over the level of access that the government can and should have to citizens' health information. This particular point, while a potential issue in any health care system, is particularly likely to arise in countries (such as Canada, Australia, and the United Kingdom) that have single-payer systems.[2]

CANADA

Canada has comprehensive data privacy laws at both the federal and state levels. At the federal level, the Personal Information Protection and Electronic Documents Act[3] (the Canadian Act) is comprehensive legislation that is intended to "govern the collection, use, and disclosure of personal information to protect the privacy of individuals" while recognizing "the need of organizations to collect, use, or disclose personal information for purposes that a reasonable person would consider appropriate in the circumstances."[4] In a guide to the Canadian Act, the Canadian Privacy Commissioner defines "personal information" as "information in any form such as: age, name, ID numbers, income, ethnic origin, or blood type; opinions, evaluations. . . ."[5] It does not, however, include "the name, title, business address, or telephone number of an employee of an organization."[6] Canadian courts have interpreted the meaning of personal information broadly and applied it to all information that presents "a serious possibility that an individual could be identified through the use of that information, alone or in combination with other information."[7] It has been applied to information that is not in written form (like video surveillance or biological samples), subjective information about an individual, and even information that is publicly available.[8]

The Canadian Act has been implemented in three phases. The first phase, which became effective in 2001, applies to certain data collected "in connection with the operation of a federal work, undertaking or business"[9] as well as to organizations that, in the course of commercial activity, disclose the personal information outside the province in exchange for consideration.[10] During Phase II, which commenced in 2002, the health care sector was required to comply with the terms of the act.[11] Finally, Phase III, which commenced in 2004, broadened the reach of the law to regulate all personal information collected, used, or disclosed in the course of all commercial activity,[12] which is defined broadly to include "any particular transaction, act, or conduct, or any regular course of conduct that is of a commercial character, including the selling, bartering or leasing of donor, membership, or other fund-raising lists."[13] With the Canadian Act entering into force in these different phases, it is significant to note that the legislation does not have any grandfather clause. As such, if entities collect personal information prior to the effective date of the act, they will not be able to use or disclose such information unless the data at issue was collected and will be used in accordance with the requirements of the Canadian Act.

The Canadian Act incorporates the Canadian Standards Association Model Code for the Protection of Personal Information, a model code that was adopted by the National Standard of Canada in 1996 (the Code).[14] Although these principles are described in the Canadian Act as recommendations, an entity's failure to comply with such recommendations can constitute grounds for a complaint. The Code and the Act are based upon 10 principles:

1. accountability;
2. identifying purposes;
3. knowledge and consent;
4. limiting collection;

5. limiting use, disclosure, and retention;
6. accuracy;
7. safeguards;
8. openness;
9. individual access; and
10. challenging compliance.

The Act places two key categories of obligations on entities: (i) obligations concerning the processing of personal information, and (ii) various administrative obligations. In terms of the substantive obligations concerning the processing of personal information, entities will be required to identify and document the limited purposes for which the personal data they collect will be processed. They will also have to ensure that they have the data subject's consent for the processing of their data for that specific identified purpose.

On the administrative side, companies will be required to designate an individual who will be in charge of the personal data, adopt policies to give effect to the Canadian Act, maintain the accuracy of the personal information, retain personal information for only as long as is necessary for the purpose of its processing, adopt security safeguards to protect personal information, provide access and rectification procedures to data subjects, and adopt procedures to respond to inquiries and complaints concerning compliance.

The Canadian Act specifies exceptions to the requirement that an organization acquire consent before collection, use, or disclosure of personal information. It also provides for exceptions to the access requirements. The following excerpts are not exhaustive but reflect some of the situations where information may be collected, used, or disclosed without knowledge and consent, and situations where access may be denied or limited. The Canadian Act stipulates that consent is not required when (i) collection of information clearly benefits the individual (who is not defined), and timely consent cannot be obtained; (ii) it is reasonable to expect that, if consent, is obtained, the availability or accuracy of the information would be compromised, and the collection is reasonable for purposes of investigating breach of an agreement or a violation of the laws of Canada or any province; (iii) the collection is solely for journalistic, artistic, or literary purposes; or (iv) the information is publicly available and is specified by the regulations.[15]

The Canadian Act also stipulates that knowledge and consent is not required when, in addition to the foregoing exceptions, the information is used (i) because the organization reasonably believes the information would be useful and is used to investigate an ongoing, past, or proposed contravention of the laws of Canada, a province, or a foreign jurisdiction; (ii) in connection with an emergency that threatens the life, health, or security of an individual; or (iii) in connection with statistical or scholarly study or research.[16] The third has certain requirements, namely that it is used for "purposes that cannot be achieved without using the information, the information is used in a manner that will ensure its confidentiality, it is impracticable to obtain consent, and the organization informs the Commissioner of the use before the information is used."[17]

The Canadian Act stipulates that knowledge and consent are not required when the information is disclosed for a number of reasons. For example, knowledge and consent is not required when the disclosure is made for the purpose of collecting a debt. Also, it is not necessary to obtain the individual's consent when his or her data is disclosed in connection with the interests of national security or in furtherance of the conservation of historical records.

The Canadian Act sets forth various exceptions to the requirement that organizations provide access to an individual's personal information. A number of the exceptions concern access to information provided to a government institution in connection with a subpoena, law enforcement investigations, or matters of national security. The Canadian Act also provides that access may be refused where (i) the information is protected by solicitor-client privilege, or (ii) if providing access would reveal confidential commercial information (and the confidential information is not severable from the requested information.)

Under the Canadian Act, complaints of privacy violations can be initiated by anyone. In practice, this means that an organization's customers, suppliers, and competitors could all be in a position to initiate complaints. The privacy commissioner is empowered to investigate all complaints under the Canadian Act and to attempt to resolve them by a number of methods, including mediation or conciliation. The privacy commissioner has very broad investigative powers. Provided that the commissioner is satisfied that there are reasonable grounds to proceed with the pursuit of a complaint, it can search and investigate entities' premises, administer oaths, and conduct interviews. Notwithstanding the powers of the privacy commissioner, individuals who contend that their rights under the Canadian Act have been violated still have recourse to the courts. Entities that violate the act are subjected to a range of penalties, including public disclosure of the information practices, fines (for which company directors, officers, and employees may be personally liable), and court-ordered damages.

In Canada, the Office of the Privacy Commissioner is very active. In addition to the commissioner dealing with the issue of violations of the act, there are numerous cases on the issue that were settled[18] or otherwise reached an early resolution.[19] The office also publishes a number of advisory and educational documents.

AUSTRALIA

Introduction to Applicable Legal Framework

Like Canada, Australia has comprehensive privacy legislation. The main legal instrument in Australia is Privacy Act 1988.[20] An amendment (Privacy Amendment [Private Sector] Act 2000) extended the operation of Privacy Act 1988 to cover the private health sector throughout Australia. Privacy Act 1988, as amended, is referred to hereinafter as the Australian Privacy Act.

The Australian Privacy Act covers a wide range of practices involving a person's private information, including (i) the need to obtain consent for the collection of health information; (ii) requirements about disclosures to be made to individuals upon collecting their information; (iii) considerations to be made before health information is shared with any third parties; (iv) information to be included in a privacy policy; (v) requirements for securing and storing information; and (vi) terms and procedures for providing individuals with the right to access their health records.

The provisions in the Australian Privacy Act are based around 10 National Privacy Principles (NPPs) that represent the minimum privacy standards for handling personal information. The 10 NPPs are (i) collection; (ii) use and disclosure; (iii) data quality; (iv) data security; (v) openness; (vi) access and correction; (vii) identifiers; (viii) anonymity; (ix) transborder data flows; and (x) sensitive information. The NPPs are quite consistent with principles that we see in other key privacy instruments, such as the European Union's Data Protection Directive.

The enforcement of the Australian Privacy Act is generally conducted through the resolution of individual complaints lodged with the Australian Privacy Commissioner. In addition, the Australian Privacy Commissioner is empowered to launch its own investigations.

The Australian Privacy Commissioner can also issue guidelines. The guidelines are advisory in nature and are designed to facilitate compliance with the requirements of the Australia Privacy Act. Of particular relevance to the current topic, in November 2001, the office of the Privacy Commissioner issued guidelines on privacy in the private health sector (Health Privacy Guidelines).[21]

Like HIPAA, the Health Privacy Guidelines apply to a limited class of entities. However, distinct from HIPAA, the Health Privacy Guidelines include a broader class of entities. Specifically, the guidelines apply to all private sector entities that provide a health service. The term "health service" is defined broadly as:

(a) An activity performed in relation to an individual that is intended or claimed (expressly or otherwise) by the individual or the person performing it: (i) to assess, record, maintain, or improve the individual's health; or (ii) to diagnose the individual's illness or disability; or (iii) to treat the individual's illness or disability or suspected illness or disability; or

b. The dispensing on prescription of a drug or medicinal preparation by a pharmacist.[22]

Thus, the Australian Health Privacy Guidelines reach typical entities such as hospitals and pharmacists, but also apply to organizations not covered by HIPAA, such as gyms and weight-loss clinics. This is a particularly interesting feature of the Australian legislation to make note of, as one of the main criticisms (and one of the most common points of misunderstanding) about HIPAA is the fact that it has a limited scope of coverage.

While the Australian Privacy Act applies to personal information, that is, information about an individual who can be identified or whose identity could be reasonably ascertained from the information, the Australian Health Privacy Guidelines apply to health information that is a subset of personal information. Health information applies only to information that is specifically about one's health, such as health services provided, information collected from a person while conducting health services, information generated by a health provider, and biological or physical information about an individual.[23] This, however, is not applicable to information that an employer holds about its current employees as long as the information and its use and disclosure relates to the employment relationship. If the information only relates to health services provided in a personal capacity, the principles still apply.[24] The principles "apply to health information held in any form, including paper, electronic, visual (x-rays, CT scans, videos, and photos), and audio records."[25]

In addition to the Australian Privacy Act and the Australian Health Privacy Guidelines, there are other commonwealth, state, and territory laws that apply to health service providers and regulate how individual health information must be handled. To the extent that there are direct inconsistencies between commonwealth and state or territory laws, generally the commonwealth law will prevail. Furthermore, the privacy of health information is protected by virtue of the obligations that health service providers have under professional and ethical codes of practice. In some instances, these codes or professional obligations apply stronger privacy protections than the Australian Privacy Act. In other respects, the Australian Privacy Act contains additional requirements to those in some professional codes of practice and may broaden the obligations of health service providers. For instance, the NPPs state that health service providers generally have to provide access to an individual to see his or her records. This right of access is an important right that is present in HIPAA and many other privacy laws. Furthermore, in addition to the general Health Privacy Guidelines, the government has also released other guidelines with potential implications for the health sector. For example, there are specific guidelines regarding the use of health information for research purposes.

Application of the Privacy Act's NPPs to the Health Sector

The following section will examine how the Privacy Act's NPPs can be applied to the health sector. It is a general, high-level summary and does not address all compliance requirements.

Principle 1: Collection

Health service providers are advised to collect only health information that is necessary for their functions or activities in treating the patient. Additionally, providers are to use fair and lawful ways to collect health information and are advised to notify data subjects as to (i) why information is being collected, (ii) to whom else the information may be disclosed, and (iii) other relevant matters, including any further disclosures required by law. Health service providers must obtain consent to collect health information, unless an exemption applies, such as where there is an emergency, it is required by law, or it relates to a legal or equitable claim.

Principle 2: Use and Disclosure

The use and disclosure principle means that organizations are to use or disclose health information solely for the primary purpose for which the information was collected unless an exception applies. There are a number of possible exceptions. For example, an organization can use the information for a secondary purpose if it is for a directly related secondary purpose within the individual's reasonable expectations. It would also be able to use or disclose the information with the data subject's consent or if there are specified law enforcement or public health and public safety circumstances.

Principle 3: Data Quality

This principle requires that health service providers take reasonable steps to ensure that all of the personal information that they are using or collecting is updated, complete, and accurate. While this principle does not mandate that health service providers continuously check all data, they must take reasonable steps to ensure its integrity. The principle of data quality, which is important in connection with all personal data, assumes particular importance in connection with medical information, since incorrect medical data can result in life-threatening medical errors.

Principle 4: Data Security

NPP 4 requires that a health service provider take reasonable steps to protect the health information it holds from misuse and loss, as well as from unauthorized access, modification, or disclosure. It also requires the provider to destroy or permanently de-identify health information that is no longer needed. The health service provider's obligation to implement safeguards applies to personal information held in several formats, such as paper, electronic form, film, photographs, audio, and video. The rationale for this principle is clear, since the failure to secure information can result in increased risk of privacy breaches, identity thefts, and other harms that have been discussed throughout this book.

Principle 5: Openness

Under the openness principle, a health service provider must have a document clearly describing its policies on the handling of personal information. It must make this document available to anyone who asks for it. It should explain what sort of personal information the provider holds, for what purposes it holds it, and the way in which it collects, holds, uses, and discloses it. Unlike HIPAA, which has very specific requirements as to the components of HIPAA, the equivalent provisions of the Australian Privacy Act give organizations a fair amount of freedom and flexibility for determining the content and format of their privacy disclosures. Still, at a minimum, the privacy policy must cover: (i) whether the health service provider is bound by the Australian Privacy Act or a code approved by the country's privacy commissioner; (ii) any exemptions or exceptions that the provider qualifies for; and (iii) that information is available upon request about the way the provider handles personal information.

In addition, health service providers in particular should also explain (i) the reason for collecting different types of information; (ii) procedures that the provider has for the collection, disclosure, or usage of the information; (iii) laws that require that the provider disclose information to other organizations; (iv) the procedures for requests for access; (v) procedures that the provider has in place to deal with breaches of privacy; and (vi) details on how to contact the provider.

Principle 6: Access and Correction

The access and correction principle establishes the health service provider's obligations regarding giving an individual access to their personal information. These include (i) giving them access to it upon request unless there are special circumstances (a serious threat to life or health and other public interest matters such as law enforcement-related issues); (ii) withholding access when it is required by law; (iii) attempting to provide access through an intermediary when access would otherwise be denied; and (iv) correcting an individual's personal information upon request.

Again, these are a lot of the same rights that exist under HIPAA. However, the Australian rules generally are far less specific than HIPAA with respect to how entities must provide access to information and the correction of information. The Australian Health Privacy Guidelines offer additional guidance on how entities should respond to requests for access and corrections, but again, these guidelines do not have the same power as law.

Principle 7: Identifiers

This principle sets out a health service provider's obligations when handling commonwealth identifiers, or numbers and codes assigned by the commonwealth to an individual to identify them for purposes of the organization's operations. Except in certain circumstances, this principle prohibits health service providers from adopting these commonwealth-issued identifiers. It does not apply to identifiers that are assigned by state or territorial government agencies (as opposed to the commonwealth, which is national). This principle also prohibits the use or disclosure of national identifiers, except when these uses or disclosures are necessary to fulfill obligations to national agencies, or when certain other provisions apply. This principle is thus similar to the growing body of legal restrictions that apply to Social Security numbers in the United States.

Principle 8: Anonymity

This principle sets out a health service provider's obligation to allow an individual to have the option of anonymity when entering transactions with the provider as long as it is lawful and practicable. Remaining anonymous or using an alias when seeking health care is an interest that many might have. This principle is designed to ensure that this can occur, except for those situations in which it may not be lawful for a provider to provide a service anonymously. This may happen, for example, if the person seeking care has a communicable disease for which the provider has reporting obligations.

Principle 9: Trans-Border Data Flows

This principle covers the obligations that a health service provider has when transferring personal information outside of Australia. The obligations only apply to transfers overseas. There are five ways that a provider can transfer personal information overseas: (i) if the provider has a reasonable belief that the recipient of the information has similar privacy schemes as Australia; (ii) if it obtained consent from the individual; (iii) if the transfer of data is necessary to complete or perform a contract made by, or in the interests of, the individual; (iv) if the transfer is for the individual's benefit and it was not practicable for the provider to obtain consent and the provider can show that if it were possible to obtain consent, the individual would be likely to give it; or (v) other reasonable steps are taken to ensure that the information is held, used, or disclosed consistently with the NPPs. Similar trans-border rules are present in European privacy laws, but there are no similar provisions in U.S. privacy laws.

Principle 10: Changes in Business Circumstances

Under this principle, a health service provider that has undergone a business change may have a duty to its patients. The duty will only arise if, as a result of the business change, the information that was collected will now be used in a way that is inconsistent with the purpose of the original collection. It is advised to obtain consent from the patient before disclosing any medical information because, of course, that is always the safest approach when disclosing one's private information, and there are times that consent would need to be obtained anyway when medical information is being transferred to another entity.

Legislative Overhaul

It is anticipated that significant changes to the Australian Privacy Act will soon be implemented. In 2008, the Australian Law Reform Commission completed a major inquiry into Australia's privacy laws and released a comprehensive report that recommended that significant changes be made to the Privacy Act.[26] The inquiry and resulting report were extremely comprehensive and addressed a number of different aspects of privacy regulation. While many of the recommendations would apply generally to all aspects of privacy, including the privacy of medical information, the report also included recommendations specifically targeted to health information. Specifically, the Australian Law Reform Commission recommended the drafting of new privacy (health information) regulations to regulate this medical privacy. The report also included recommendations concerning electronic[27] health records and to address greater facilitation of health and medical research. In 2009, the Australian government committed to implementing a large number of recommendations that the Australian Law Reform Commission had made in its comprehensive report.[28] Accordingly, it is anticipated that we will see significant changes to Australian privacy laws in the near future.

THE EUROPEAN APPROACH

Introduction to Privacy in the EU

There are a number of important laws applicable to privacy in the European Union. Key among them is the European Data Protection Directive (the Data Protection Directive),[29] which was passed on October 24, 1995, and came into effect on October 25, 1998. It is extremely comprehensive legislation that concerns all aspects of personal data processing. It treats the protection of personal data from a very broad perspective. Indeed, "personal data" is defined very broadly under the directive as "any information relating to an identified or identifiable natural person."[30]

The Data Protection Directive, as other European Community directives, is not a law directed at individual entities. Instead, it serves as a set of directions to the member states of the European Union requiring them to implement certain requirements in their own national laws. The result of this is that while the laws of each member state are required to be consistent with the directive, they will often differ from each other in certain potentially significant ways. This is a significant detail because entities in control of operations involving the processing of personal data (also called controllers) must comply with the data-protection laws of the country in which they are established, as well as the laws of the particular member state(s) in which they process personal data.[31] While the Data Protection Directive is intended to ensure that the free market functions correctly, the liberty that individual member states have in implementing it means that there will be significant compliance obligations from state to state.

Basic Principles

The directive addresses the protection of personal data from a number of different perspectives. At its most basic level, it establishes certain conditions that must be met in order to process personal data. It specifies that there are only six situations pursuant to which entities can process personal data:

(i) The individual has provided his or her unambiguous consent to such processing;

(ii) The individual has entered into a contract that provides for, or anticipates, the processing of the data;

(iii) The processing is necessary to fulfill a legal obligation of the individual;

(iv) The processing is necessary to protect the individual's "vital interests";

(v) The processing is in the public interest, or is being done at the behest of an official authority; or

(vi) The processing is necessary to pursue the legitimate interests of the party collecting or using the data, except to the extent that those interests may be overridden by the rights of the individual to the privacy of the information about himself/herself.[32]

In addition to these general preconditions that are applicable to all kinds of personal data, the Data Protection Directive places heightened restrictions on the collection and use of "special categories" of personal data, which consists of "personal data revealing racial or ethnic origin, political opinions, religious or philosophical beliefs, trade union membership, and the processing of data concerning health or sex life."[33] These special categories of data may only be processed if:

(i) The individual has provided his or her consent, provided that the laws of the particular member states recognize it;

(ii) The party collecting or using the information is doing so in fulfillment of its legal employment law-related obligations;

(iii) The individual is unable to give consent, and his or her vital interests are at stake;

(iv) The party collecting or using the information is a nonprofit organization with a political, philosophical, religious, or trade union aim of which the individual is a member or is regularly associated;

(v) The information is the subject of legal claims or has otherwise been made public;

(vi) The information concerns health care, provided it is collected or used by a professional under a legal or professional obligation of confidentiality; or

(vii) Such use or collection of data is in the interest of substantial public interest in accordance with national law.[34]

Notice Requirements

The Data Protection Directive also has significant notice requirements. Under its terms, entities processing personal data must notify the applicable data-protection supervisory authorities of the details of their data-processing operations of the member state in which they are operating.[35] The supervisory authority of each member state tends to have its own procedural and notice requirements. However, generally the notice that is made to the supervisory authorities must indicate:

(a) The name and address of the controller and of his representative, if any;

(b) The purpose or purposes of the processing;

(c) A description of the category or categories of the data subject and of the data or categories of data relating to them;

(d) The recipients or categories of recipient to whom the data might be disclosed;

(e) Proposed transfers of data to third countries; and

(f) A general description allowing a preliminary assessment to be made of the appropriateness of the measures taken pursuant to Article 17 to ensure the security of processing.[36]

The notice requirements are very important. In many countries, failing to act in accordance with the notice requirements can leave the controller subject to serious penalties. The notice requirements play a very important role in the overall scheme of personal data protection. The intent of the comprehensive notice requirements appears to be to ensure that the individual who is the subject of data-processing operations can effectively monitor the movement of his or her personal data as it moves between different data processors and data controllers.

The Rights of the Data Subject

The directive provides individuals who are data subjects with significant rights to ensure that the entity that is controlling the processing of their data is not processing more personal data than is necessary and is processing the correct data. Specifically, pursuant to the terms of the directive, data subjects have the right to obtain the following information from the data controller:

(i) Whether the controller has any data about the individual;

(ii) The purpose for which the data is being used, if any;

(iii) The categories of data that have been obtained;

(iv) The recipients or categories of recipients of the data;

(v) The actual data undergoing processing, in a readable form;

(vi) The source of the data, if known; and

(vii) To the extent the data is being used in any "automated decision-making" capacity, and the logic by which such decisions are being made.[37]

The directive requires that such information be provided to the data subject "without constraint" and "without excessive delay or expense."[38] Such rights of access and rectification, not generally available in the United States, appear to be a very important part of ensuring that personal data is used properly and in compliance with the applicable law. If access and rectification rights are truly available and are actually used by data subjects, the likelihood that incorrect data will linger in organizations' systems diminishes substantially.

Data Security

The directive also requires data controllers and processors to implement appropriate security measures to protect personal data. This obligation, which is meant to ensure that personal data is afforded adequate security, is a requirement that is appearing in an increasing number of laws and regulations both in the United States and abroad. When analyzed, the requirement is very logical. In reality, entities' promises concerning the limitations on the use and transfer of personal data that they collect are only as useful as the security measures that they implement to protect such data.

The Data Protection Directive establishes a relatively broad and general rule concerning the security of personal data, providing:

Member states shall provide that the controller must implement appropriate technical and organizational measures to protect personal data against accidental or unlawful destruction or accidental loss and against unauthorized alteration, disclosure or access, in particular where the processing involves the transmission of data over a network, and against all other unlawful forms of processing.[39]

Further, in determining what security measures would be "appropriate," the directive calls upon data controllers to consider the state of the available technology, the cost of the implementation of the security measures, the risks represented by the processing, and the nature of the data to be protected.[40]

The result of the use of such general language in the directive is that there are considerable differences in the security requirements—and the penalties for violating those requirements—from member state to member state. Many member states have implemented stringent requirements that may vary somewhat based upon the kind of processing that is being undertaken. In Spain, for example, entities that process health information are obliged to comply with more stringent data security requirements than they are when processing other personal data.[41]

It is also notable that the European approach to data security seeks to hold the controller accountable for the security measures that are implemented by any third party data processors involved with the processing of personal data. Under the terms of the directive, controllers are not able to simply delegate their security obligations to the processing entities. Instead, the directive compels controllers who rely on data processors to "choose a processor providing sufficient guarantees in respect of the technical security measures and organizational measures governing the processing to be carried out. . ."[42] Furthermore, the directive requires the controller and processor to enter into an agreement that binds the processor to the controller and stipulates that the processor may only act upon the instructions of the controller and that the processor must act in compliance with the security requirements of the directive as they are implemented in the laws of the relevant member state(s).[43]

Cross-Border Data Transfers

One of the most notable aspects of the Data Protection Directive is the section concerning transfers of personal data to countries outside of the European Economic Area. The directive prohibits the transfer of personal data to third countries that do not provide adequate protection of personal data unless one of several limited exceptions applies.[44]

The directive sets forth a list of factors to be taken into account when judging the adequacy of protection in third countries.[45] In determining whether a particular jurisdiction provides adequate protection to personal data, European authorities are required to assess not only the actual privacy laws in place in the country at issue, but also the efficacy of those laws.

Significant in relation to making adequacy assessments is the working party that was established pursuant to Article 29 of the Data Protection Directive (the Working Party) and which is composed of data protection commissioners from each EU member state along with European Commission officials. The Working Party has produced useful guidance documents on the approaches that are to be taken when evaluating whether the level of protection provided in a third country is adequate.[46] The approach put forth by the Working Party focuses on a set of principles. The first principle is the purpose-limitation principle. According to this principle, personal data should be processed for a specific purpose and subsequently used or further communicated only insofar as this process is compatible with the purpose of the transfer.

The second principle is the data quality and proportionality principle. According to this principle, data should be accurate and, where necessary, kept up-to-date. Furthermore, personal data should be adequate, relevant, and not excessive in relation to the purposes for which they are transferred or further processed.

The transparency principle is the third principle. In accordance with this principle, individuals should be provided with information as to the purpose of the processing and the identity of the data controller in the third country and other information insofar as this information is necessary to ensure fairness.

Next is the security principle. Pursuant to this principle, technical and organizational security measures should be taken that are appropriate to the risks presented by the processing. Any person acting under the authority of the data controller must not process data except upon instruction from the data controller.

The individual's rights to access, rectification, and opposition must also be considered. According to this principle, the data subject should have a right to obtain a copy of all data relating to him or her that are processed and a right to rectification of those data where they are shown to be inaccurate. In certain situations, he or she should also be able to object to the processing of the data relating to him or her.

Finally, restrictions on onward transfers must also be considered. Generally, transfers of personal data from the recipient to another third party should not be permitted unless a means is found contractually binding the third party in question, thereby providing the same data protection guarantees to the data subjects. This principle is important in relation to the European regulators' intent to prohibit the use of countries with "adequate" protection as intermediaries for exporting data to the actual destination country where such destination country does not provide adequate protection of personal data.

To date, the European Commission has approved of only a small number of jurisdictions, including Hungary, Switzerland, Canada, Argentina,

Jersey, and Guernsey as providing adequate protection of personal data. The Article 29 Working Party recently opined that Andorra and Israel offer adequate protection of personal data and it is anticipated that an official commission decision will follow shortly. Of course, the U.S. Safe Harbors program has also been deemed to constitute adequate protection of personal data. Entities that desire to participate in the Safe Harbors Program must certify that they comply with the seven major principles of the initiative, which are notice, choice, onward transfer, access, security, data integrity, and enforcement.

Working Party Guidance on Electronic Health Records

In 2007, the Working Party put together a working document to provide guidance on data-protection principles in relation to electronic health records (EHRs).[47] The Working Party prepared this working document in response to the concern about how the use of EHRs can impact an individual's privacy. The working document is based on the Data Protection Directive and sets forth several principles that one must comply with in relation to EHRs.

The working document advises that more stringent rules should apply to EHRs than "ordinary" personal data. The working document reminds us that EHRs would be categorized as "sensitive personal data" under the directive and therefore subject to the rules set forth in Article 8 of the directive. The general rule for sensitive information under the directive is that it cannot be processed when it relates to one's health in general. There are several exceptions to the rule. One is when the data subject gives "explicit consent" to the processing of the data, which includes the data subject being aware of the sensitivity of the information. The consent must be voluntary, specific (on a specific situation, not general consent), and informed (everything must be given in a clear and understandable manner). Another exception is when the individual cannot give consent and the processing is necessary to protect his or her vital interests. Another exception is when the processing of the sensitive data is required for a specific medical purpose (preventative medicine, diagnoses, etc.) and it is done by a medical professional under the rules of that country. In addition to the exceptions, the directive also allows a member state to derogate from the prohibition when there is a substantial public interest to allow the processing of the data and there are suitable safeguards in place to protect the fundamental rights and privacy of individuals. A substantial interest would include things that relate to social security interests and public health interests.

Beyond applying the rules of the directive to EHRs, the working document also provided recommendations on the following 11 topics where special safeguards within EHR systems seem particularly necessary in order to guarantee the data protection rights of patients and individuals: (i) respecting self determination; (ii) identification and authentication of patients and health care professionals; (iii) authorization for accessing EHRs in order to read and write in EHRs; (iv) use of EHRs for other purposes; (v) organizational structure of an EHR system; (vi) categories of data stored in EHRs and modes of their presentation; (vii) international transfer of medical records; (viii) data security; (ix) transparency; (x) liability issues; and (xi) control mechanisms for processing data in EHRs.[48]

Subsequent to the issuance of the working document, the European Commission launched major initiatives aimed at achieving interoperable e-health systems across Europe.[49] Among other goals, the initiatives are intended to facilitate the availability of electronic health records across national borders.

CONCLUSION

Many individuals consider information about their health and medical status to be among the most private and confidential information about themselves. It is thus little wonder that most countries have strong legislative measures in place to protect the privacy of health information. There are, however, as has been demonstrated in this chapter, a variety of ways in which lawmakers can and have strived to protect the privacy, security, and confidentiality of this most sensitive information.

As privacy continues to face ever-growing risks and continuously transforming threats, it is wise to consider some of the efforts underway in other jurisdictions when evaluating whether our current laws are sufficient. For example, laws in place in Canada and throughout the European Union take a broad and holistic view of privacy protection. Whereas HIPAA only applies to certain types of entities and information, these omnibus privacy laws have a much broader reach and there appears to be great value in this. Given the legal framework presently in place in the United States, an entity that collects your medical information but that is not subject to HIPAA, such as perhaps a spa or gym, would not have the same privacy and security obligations as your doctor. Once an entity receives medical information from or about you, shouldn't that entity be required to protect the privacy and security of that information? Is it really fair to say that because the entity does not fall into the limited class of entities that are regulated by HIPAA, they should not have the same obligations as the covered entities do? A review of some of the approaches taken in these other countries begs these very questions. While HIPAA does require certain entities to provide comprehensive protections to the privacy and security of medical information, it remains questionable as to whether that is truly enough. Considering the omnibus regimes in place

Conclusion

OVERVIEW

Patient privacy is integral to proper medical care and the respect of human dignity. Fortunately, it is a concept that is well engrained in our health care traditions. The principle of doctor-patient confidentiality goes back to ancient times. This inviolable principle can in fact be traced back to the fourth century BCE, originating with the Hippocratic Oath, and it remains sacrosanct to the present day. The importance of the duty of confidentiality in the present day is recognized in the American Medical Association's Code of Medical Ethics.[1] Across the globe, health care providers treat patients with a recognition of and a deep appreciation for this fundamental duty.

In recent years, technological innovations and transformations in the business of medicine have led to significant changes in the delivery of health care and have increased the proliferation of private medical information. Today, your medical information can be accessed by a wide range of individuals beyond your direct health care provider. Furthermore, from health researchers, to marketers, to your employer, even to your curious acquaintances and family members, a great number of constituencies have an interest in your medical information. This all translates to enhanced risks to privacy and security of your medical information. In light of this new environment, this book has endeavored to highlight the current threats to your privacy, inform you about the protections available to you under existing law, identify deficiencies in the current legal environment, and provide you with the tools you need to better protect yourself. Before closing this discussion, I offer a few suggestions on how we, as a nation, may improve the privacy protections currently available under law, and, perhaps more significantly, I offer some final suggestions on steps you can take to protect your own health privacy.

IMPROVING PRIVACY PROTECTIONS

In examining the current legal framework applicable to medical privacy, this book has not only explored the protections offered by existing laws, but it has also highlighted their limitations. To be equipped to play a role in protecting and defending our own health privacy, we must first understand the extent to which existing laws do and do not protect us.

As discussed throughout this book, medical privacy is protected by a number of important laws, as well as, at least insofar as medical providers are concerned, professional duties of confidentiality. Still, as society, technology, and health care services continue to evolve, our medical privacy will face new threats. In addition, existing threats to health privacy can become more serious and/or can overcome the protections that we have developed against those threats.

As outlined below, there are several key issues upon which the emphasis of reform efforts should be placed.

Data Security: Proper data security is fundamental to privacy. If private health information is not kept secure from unauthorized access, use, and/or disclosure, the patient's privacy interests in that information will be lost. The patient can then suffer a number of negative consequences, including possible discrimination and emotional distress. The patient may even become the victim of identity theft and experience the financial losses that this often entails. The importance of data security goes far beyond this, however. Quality health care depends upon access to accurate, reliable, and complete medical information. Inadequate data security raises the risks that health information may be altered or destroyed, thereby compromising patient safety and care. The HIPAA Privacy Rule goes pretty far in protecting data security, and the recent extension of the application of the HIPAA Privacy Rule to business associates should also help to improve security. However, additional improvements can be made. For instance, consideration should be directed toward understanding whether encryption should be mandatory. In addition, recall that the HIPAA Privacy Rule does not apply to paper-based documents. While the risks to electronic data may be more serious, paper-based information can remain vulnerable to security threats.

Extension of privacy rights to entities beyond covered entities: As discussed in Chapter 8, many foreign countries that have enacted laws to protect privacy have implemented omnibus privacy laws that protect all personal data, irrespective of what industry is involved and what kind of entity is collecting, using, or sharing the information. Moreover, beyond the stringent baseline privacy protections that apply to all data, in many of these jurisdictions, even more protective rules apply to "special" or "sensitive" data, a category that will almost always include medical information. In contrast, for the most part, in the United States, privacy laws are based upon particular industrial sectors, and our health privacy laws are directed to a relatively limited class of entities: covered entities, and to a certain, but increasing, extent, their business associates. Given the fact that these are not the only types of companies that may have access to your medical information, should we not consider an approach that would ensure a certain level of protection for all health-related information, irrespective of the type of entity that is using it?

Greater patient education: Even though HIPAA has been in place for many years now, there continues to be a high level of misunderstanding about what HIPAA does and does not do. Some people believe that they have greater rights under HIPAA than they actually do. Also, many people are unaware of how they may exercise the rights that they have. While legislators have attempted to increase individual awareness by requiring the circulation of detailed HIPAA Privacy Notices, there are real questions as to whether this is adequate. It seems that few people read the notices and even when they are read, they are often misunderstood. There is a real movement for the use of more plain language in privacy notices. Such an effort is currently underway in connection with the privacy notices that are to be issued by financial institutions under the Gramm-Leach-Bliley Act and, as one means of improving patient education, we may also wish to consider a similar approach with respect to the notices that are issued under HIPAA.

Investigation into de-identification risks: As outlined in Chapter 6, recent attention has been directed to understanding the risks of de-identified data. In the recent past, it was largely assumed that if data were properly de-identified, there would be few risks involved with permitting the widespread disclosure and use of that data. However, there is increasing evidence that de-identified data may not be as anonymous as once believed. At the same time, however, important medical research often hinges upon the use of de-identified data. Further investigation is needed to understand the extent to which current methods of de-identification protect the privacy of patient data and to understand what changes may be necessary. The recent HHS workshops on this topic were a great first step, but additional study is needed.

PROTECTING YOURSELF

Even if the existing legal frameworks applicable to medical privacy were perfect, we would all still have a role to play in protecting our own health privacy. After all, we cannot disclose intimate details about our medical history in public forums on the Web and expect that the information will be private and confidential. Beyond limiting your public disclosures of privacy health matters, as discussed below, there are a number of steps that you can take in order to improve the likelihood that the personal medical information that you wish to protect as private will remain so.

Educate yourself: Find out as much as you can about the privacy practices of your health care provider and health plan. Read the covered entity's notice of privacy practices and make sure that you understand it. Ask questions if you do not understand the notice or want any other information about your provider's policies and practices.

Protect your own information: Protect the privacy of your Social Security number and other personal information. Disclose to your physician all information that may be needed for your diagnosis and medical care; however, think twice about disclosing anything that may not be remotely related to your health, as this can end up being part of your medical record.

Communicate: Talk to your health care provider about any confidentiality concerns that you may have. Ask how the provider shares patient data within the office and with affiliates.

Stay informed: Ask to review your medical records before your doctor sends them to a third party such as an insurer. Ask to be notified if your medical records are ever subpoenaed.

Shop around: You are not only a patient, but also a consumer of medical services, and like any consumer, you can shop for the best deal around in terms of privacy and security protection. Of course, where your health is concerned, it will be essential to choose the best medical provider. However, it is reasonable to consider privacy and security considerations as part of your analysis.

Read authorizations carefully and make sure that you understand what you are agreeing to before signing: Make your choices about restrictions on authorizations known, and refuse to sign any you are not comfortable with. Keep in mind, authorization forms may ask for your permission in order to disclose your PHI for multiple purposes. One type of authorization is the use of your medical data for marketing. You may withdraw your authorization if you later decide you made the wrong choice. Because HIPAA authorizes so many different types of disclosures without patient approval, you should be suspicious anytime someone asks you to sign an authorization form for disclosure of PHI. Make sure that the authorization is for your benefit and not for the benefit of someone else.

Exercise your right to obtain a copy of your medical records: Make sure that your PHI is accurate. Request that incorrect information be corrected or amended. However, keep in mind that your health care provider has the final word on changes and amendments to health records.

Keep a personal health record: This may include copies of your medical files and other information related to your health, such as any wellness programs in which you may participate. However, if you do use a PHR, make sure to remain mindful of the risk-mitigation strategies discussed in Chapter 4.

Request that communications from your providers be made in a way that you choose: For example, you can request that you be called on your cell phone rather than your home phone, or that mailings be sent to your P.O. Box rather than your residential address.

Be wary of promotions and offers that are too good to be true: They probably are and they may be a means for fraudsters to get your information that they can then use for identity theft and other harm.

Exercise your right to file a complaint: If you feel your rights have been violated or your concerns have been ignored, you can file a complaint with both the provider and the HHS Office of Civil Rights. Many problems can be resolved by going directly to the health care provider before you contact HHS.

Understand the trade-offs before agreeing to marketing initiatives: Popular promotions, including the use of supermarket and pharmacy discount cards, can result in unexpected uses of your personal information. For some, the advantages of promotions will far outweigh any perceived privacy risks. For others, however, the potential privacy concerns may be considered to be much more significant than any financial benefits from the promotion. The key point will be to ensure that you understand the terms of the promotion and what, if anything, you are giving up by accepting it. Also, if you are not interested in receiving unsolicited marketing offers, as discussed in Chapter 6, make sure to remove yourself from marketing lists.

Exercise discretion: In the contemporary era, there is a great tendency toward disclosure. However, if you would like for your information to be private, you must exercise discretion in choosing what information you choose to disclose and to whom.

Glossary of Select Terms

ARRA: The American Reinvestment and Recovery Act of 2009.

Business associate: A business associate is, with respect to a covered entity, a person who on behalf of such covered entity or of an organized health care arrangement in which the covered entity participates, but other than in the capacity of a member of the workforce of such covered entity or arrangement, performs, or assists in the performance of: (a) a function or activity involving the use or disclosure of individually identifiable health information, including claims processing or administration, data analysis, processing or administration, utilization review, quality assurance, billing, benefit management, practice management, and repricing; (b) any other function or activity regulated by the HIPAA Privacy Rule; or (c) provides, other than in the capacity of a member of the workforce of such covered entity, legal, actuarial, accounting, consulting, data aggregation, management, administrative, accreditation, or financial services to or for such covered entity, or to or for an organized health care arrangement in which the covered entity participates, where the provision of the service involves the disclosure of individually identifiable health information from such covered entity or arrangement, or from another business associate of such covered entity or arrangement, to the person.[1]

CMS: The Centers for Medicare & Medicaid Services within the Department of Health & Human Services.

Covered entity: Covered entities are health plans, health care clearinghouses, and health care providers who transmit health information in electronic form in connection with transactions covered by HIPAA.

Disclosure: The release, transfer, provision of, access to, or divulging in any other manner of information outside the entity holding the information.

Electronic health record: An electronic version of a patient's medical history that is maintained by the provider over time and may include all of the key administrative clinical data relevant to that person's care under a particular provider, including demographics, progress notes, problems, medications, vital signs, past medical history, immunizations, laboratory data, and radiology reports

FTC: The Federal Trade Commission.

Health plan: An individual or group plan that provides or pays the cost of medical care.

HHS: The Department of Health & Human Services.

HIPAA: The Health Insurance Portability and Accountability Act.

HIT: Health information technology.

HITECH Act: The Health Information Technology for Economic and Clinical Health Act.

Individually identifiable health information: Individually identifiable health information is information that is a subset of health information, including demographic information collected from an individual and (1) is created or received by a health care provider, health plan, employer, or health care clearinghouse; and (2) relates to the past, present, or future physical or mental health or condition of an individual; the provision of health care to an individual; or the past, present, or future payment for the provision of health care to an individual; and (i) identifies the individual; or (ii) with respect to which there is a reasonable basis to believe the information can be used to identify the individual.

Medical ID theft: Medical identity theft occurs when an identity thief uses personal identifiers such as a Social Security number of a victim to obtain medical care, services, products, insurance benefits, or insurance.

Medical privacy: Medical privacy can mean different things to different people (just as the concept of privacy itself can). However, as explained in the original HIPAA Privacy Rule, the right of individuals to medical privacy means the right to determine for themselves when, how, and to what extent information about them is communicated.

The Patient Protection and Affordable Care Act (PPACA) of 2010: The PPACA is the major health insurance reform package that was signed into law on March 23, 2010.

Personal health record, or PHR: A health record concerning a consumer that includes medical information from a number of different sources (such as the consumer, an insurance carrier, doctors, and laboratories) that is established and maintained by the consumer, often online via the Internet.

PIPEDA: The Personal Information Protection and Electronic Documents Act, the key federal privacy legislation in Canada.

Protected health information, or PHI: Identifiable health information about individuals that is created or received by a health plan, provider, or health care clearinghouse and is transmitted or maintained in any form.

Use: Use means, with respect to individually identifiable health information, the sharing, employment, application, utilization, examination, or analysis of such information within an entity that maintains it.

Notes

INTRODUCTION

1. Hippocratic Oath, http://www.nlm.nih.gov/hmd/greek/greek_oath.html (accessed May 18, 2010).

2. *Olmstead v. United States*, 277 U.S. 438, 478 (1928) (Brandeis, J., dissenting); Samuel D. Warren and Louis D. Bradeis, "The Right to Privacy," 4 *Harvard Law Review* 193 (1890).

3. Symposium, "Privacy As Contextual Integrity," 79 *Wash. L. Rev.* 119 (2004).

4. Symposium, "Personal Privacy and Common Goods: A Framework for Balancing Under the National Health Information Privacy Rule," 86 *Minn. L. Rev.* 1439 (2002).

5. California Health Care Foundation: "Medical Privacy and Confidentiality Survey (1999)," http://www.chcf.org/topics/view.cfm?itemID=12500 (accessed February 15, 2010).

6. Steven Greenhouse and Martin Barbaro, "Wal-Mart Memo Suggests Ways to Cut Employee Benefit Costs, *New York Times*, October 26, 2005, http://www.nytimes.com/2005/10/26/business/26walmart.ready.html(accessed August 21, 2010) (discussing a memorandum circulated by Walmart's executive vice president for benefits, suggesting that discouraging unhealthy job applicants would be an efficient way to cut employee benefit costs).

7. Melissa Weddle and Patricia K. Kokotailo, "Confidentiality and Consent in Adolescent Substance Abuse: An Update," *AMA J. Ethics*, March 2005, http://virtualmentor.ama-assn.org/2005/03/pfor1-0503.html (accessed February 15, 2010).

8. Medical Records Confidentiality: Issues Affecting the Mental Health and Substance Abuse Systems, posting of John Petrila to Med-Privacy@essential.org (April 28, 1999).

9. Janssen, R. S., Holtgrave, D. R., Valdiserri, R. O., Shepherd, M., Gayle, H., DeCock, K. M. "The Serostatus Approach to Fighting the HIV Epidemic: prevention strategies for infected individuals." *American Journal of Public Health.* 2001; 91:1019–1024.

10. Terry, N. P., and Francis, L. P., "Ensuring the Privacy and Confidentiality of Electronic Health Records," 2007 *U. Ill. L. Rev* 681; see also Adam D. Moore, "Intangible Property: Privacy, Power and Information Control," 35 *Am. Philosophical Q.* 365 (1998).

11. Universal Declaration of Human Rights, G.A. Res. 217A, at 73, U.N. GAOR, 3d Sess., 1st plen. mtg., U.N. Doc. A/810 (December 10, 1948). Article 12 of the Universal Declaration of Human Rights provides: "No one shall be subjected to arbitrary interference with his privacy, family, home or correspondence, nor to attacks upon his honour and reputation. Everyone has the right to the protection of the law against such interference or attacks." Id.

12. Health Insurance Portability and Accountability Act (HIPAA), 42 U.S.C. 201 (2006).

13. California Health Care Foundation, Health Privacy, National Consumer Health Privacy Survey 2005, http://www.chcf.org/topics/view.cfm?itemID=115694 (accessed February 18, 2010).

14. PatientPrivacyRights.org, "UPI Poll: Concern on Health Privacy (2007)," http://patientprivacyrights.org/2007/02/upi-poll-concern-on-health-privacy/ (accessed August 21, 2010).

15. HarrisInteractive.com, "Harris Poll #74: Millions Believe Personal Medical Information Has Been Lost or Stolen (2008)," http://harrisinteractive.com/harris_poll/index.asp?PID=930 (accessed February 19, 2010).

16. Declan McCullagh, "U.S. Stimulus Bill Pushes e-Health Records for All," CNET News, February 10, 2009, http://news.cnet.com/8301-13578_3-10161233-38.html (discusses how the 2009 stimulus legislation encourages the adoption of electronic health records); see also Robert Pear, "Privacy Issue Complicates Push to Link Medical Data," *New York Times*, January 17, 2009, http://www.nytimes.com/2009/01/18/us/politics/18health.html (discusses the privacy implications of electronic health records).

17. Schulte, F., "Stimulus Fuels Gold Rush For Electronic Health Systems," Huffington Post, November 9, 2009, http://www.huffingtonpost.com/2009/11/05/stimulus-fuels-gold-rush_n_347311.html (accessed March 11, 2010).

18. Id.

19. Brody, J. E., "Medical Paper Trail Takes Electronic Turn," *New York Times*, February 22, 2010, http://www.nytimes.com/2010/02/23/health/23brod.html (discusses some of the advantages and disadvantages of a transition to electronic health records) (accessed March 11, 2010).

20. Schulte, F., and Schwartz, E., "Experts: Move To Electronic Medical Records Needs Oversight," Huffington Post, February 25, 2010, http://www.huffingtonpost.com/2010/ 02/25/experts-move-to-electroni_n_477546.html (notes that "[e]arlier this week, the U.S. Food and Drug Administration disclosed that potential safety risks from health information technology—including reports of six patient deaths and

several dozen injuries in the past two years—have prompted it to lay out proposals for regulating the devices for the first time"); see also Wangsness, L. "Electronic Health Records Raise Doubt," *Boston Globe*, April 13, 2009, http://www.boston.com/news/nation/washington/articles/2009/04/13/electronic_health_records_raise_doubt/discussing one individual's experience with medical errors in his personal health record) (accessed March 11, 2010).

21. Moore, E. A. "E-prescriptions More Reliable Than Handwritten Ones," CNET News, February 26, 2010, http://news.cnet.com/8301-27083_3-10460672-247.html (discussing recent research at Weill Cornell Medical College in New York that demonstrated that medical professionals writing prescriptions by hand are seven times more likely to make errors than those using electronic systems).

22. American Recovery and Reinvestment Act, Pub. L. No. 111-5, 123 Stat. 115 (2009).

23. Health Information Technology for Economic and Clinical Health Act, 123 Stat. at 226.

CHAPTER 1

1. Edelstein, L., *The Hippocratic Oath: Text, Translation, and Interpretation* Baltimore: Johns Hopkins Press, 1943.

2. Office of Technology Assessment, "Protecting Privacy in Computerized Medical Information," No. 576 (1993).

3. Health Insurance Portability and Accounting Act of 1996, Pub. L. No. 104-191, 110 Stat. 1936 (codified as amended in scattered sections of 42 U.S.C.).

4. Department of Health, Education and Welfare (now, Department of Health and Human Services), "Records, Computers and the Rights of Citizens: Report of the Secretary's Advisory Committee on Automated Personal Data Systems," http://aspe.hhs.gov/datacncl/1973privacy/c3.htm (accessed January 16, 2009).

5. Id.

6. Id.

7. Organization of Economic Co-operation & Development, "OECD Guidelines on the Protection of Privacy and Transborder Flows of Personal Data," September 23, 1980, http://www.oecd.org/document/18/0,2340,en_2649_34255_181518 6_1_1_1_1,00.html, (accessed March 1, 2010).

8. HIPAA Privacy Rule, 45 C.F.R. §§160;164(A); §164(E) (2009).

9. Throughout this book, there will be references to medical information, health information, protected health information, and PHI. For the most part, the terms "protected health information" and "PHI" will be used when speaking of HIPAA, whereas other terms, such as "medical information" and "health information," may be used when speaking of concepts of health privacy more generally.

10. Id. at §164.512. The following categories are all contained in this section.

11. Id. at §164.530. The following categories are all contained in this section.

12. Id. at §160.103.

13. HIPAA Security Rule, 45 C.F.R. §§164.302–164.309 (2009).

14. Office of the Inspector General, Department of Health and Human Services, A-04-07-05064, Nationwide Review of the Centers for Medicare and Medicaid

Services Health Insurance Portability and Accountability Act of 1996 Oversight (2008).

15. "HHS, Providence Health Agree on Corrective Action Plan to Protect Health Information," http://www.hhs.gov/ocr/privacy/hipaa/enforcement/examples/provi-denceresolutionagreement.html (accessed March 15, 2010).

16. Johnson, R. A. "The HIPAA Security Rule: CMS' Enforcement Activities Acquire Teeth," http://www.carf.org/consumer.aspx?content=content/About/Partners/SecurityRule.htm (accessed March 16, 2010).

17. American Recovery and Reinvestment Act, Pub. L. No. 111-5, 123 Stat. 115 (2009).

18. Health Information Technology for Economic and Clinical Health Act, 123 Stat. at 226.

19. Id. at 262.

20. Id. at 258.

21. Green, K. J., "The Benefits of Changing Times: Health Plan Compliance in 2010," 57 Fed. Law. 36, 38 (2010).

22. FTC Health Breach Notification Rule, 16 C.F.R. pt. 318 (2009).

23. The company, MedicAlert, provides such a service. http://www.medicalert.org/ (accessed March 4, 2010).

24. 74 Fed. Reg. 42,962, 42,976 (August 25, 2009) (codified at 16 C.F.R. pt. 318).

25. "[T]he Commission has brought 26 law enforcement actions since 2001 against companies that allegedly failed to maintain  reasonable procedures to protect consumers' personal information," FTC.gov, "FTC Testifies on Data Security, Peer-to-Peer File Sharing," http://www.ftc.gov/opa/2009/05/peer2peer.shtm, May 5, 2009 (accessed March 16, 2010). These actions were based on violations of different restrictions imposed by the FTC.

26. Id. at 42,740.

27. Privacy Act of 1974, 5 U.S.C. §552a (2006).

28. 42 C.F.R. pt. 2 (2009).

29. Family Educational Rights and Privacy Act, 20 U.S.C. §1232g (2006).

30. Americans with Disabilities Act, 42 U.S.C. § 12,101 (2006).

31. Genetic Information Nondiscrimination Act of 2008, Pub. L. No. 110-233, 122 Stat. 881.

32. Katz, G., and Schweitzer, S. O., "Implications of Genetic Testing for Health Policy," 10 *Yale J. Health Pol'y L. & Ethics* 90, 94 (2010).

33. I have my own recent experience on this area. After suffering from some gastrointestinal problems, my physician suggested an endoscopy to test for celiac disease. While concerned about the possibility of this ailment, I wished to avoid, or at least delay an invasive procedure. After doing some research, I found that there was a pretty strong genetic link to celiac disease and, although there continues to be some debate on this, the available research seems to suggest that one would not be likely to develop celiac disease without the presence of certain genes. Accordingly, before undergoing the endoscopy, I procured my own genetic test. It was a simple and relatively inexpensive procedure that involved taking a swab of my cheek and mailing

in the sample to a laboratory. The results were made available to me via the Internet within a few weeks. Of course, everyone should follow the advice of their physician. This example is not meant to suggest that anyone should dismiss their doctor's advice and procure their own tests. It is meant only as an example of how these kinds of genetic tests are being used. Many individuals with a family history of certain types of cancers, including, most notably breast cancer, are also seeking out these genetic tests to get an understanding of their likelihood of developing cancer.

34. 45 C.F.R. §160.203(a) (2009).

35. Id. at §160.202.

CHAPTER 2

1. Health Insurance Portability and Accounting Act of 1996, Pub. L. No. 104-191, 110 Stat. 1936 (codified as amended in scattered sections of 42 U.S.C.).

2. Siegel, K. M., Comment, "Protecting the Most Valuable Corporate Asset: Electronic Data, Identity Theft, Personal Information and the Role of Data Security in the Information Age," 111 *Penn St. L. Rev.* 779, 819 (2007) (citing Jody Westby, International Guide to Privacy [American Bar Association, 2004]). Westby argues that, "HIPAA security rules cause confusion and suggest[s] that regulators need to better understand cyber security before enacting regulations of this type." Id. at n. 226.

3. HIPAA Privacy Rule, 45 C.F.R. §§160;164(A); §164(E) (2009).

4. For more information on one's right of access to PHI, see, HIPAA Privacy Rule, 45 C.F.R. at §164.526.

5. CLIA is the abbreviation for the Clinical Laboratory Improvement Amendments. Additional information is available at http://www.cms.hhs.gov/clia (accessed March 18, 2010).

6. HIPAA Privacy Rule, 45 C.F.R. at §164.524.

7. HITECH Act, Pub. L. No. 111-5, 123 Stat. 226 (2009).

8. 45 N.Y. Pub. Health L., §18(2) (McKinney, 2004).

9. For more information on one's right to amend PHI, see HIPAA Privacy Rule, 45 C.F.R. at §164.526.

10. The request to provide a Social Security number is a thorny issue, due to the fact that Social Security numbers can be used to commit identity theft. A number of states have enacted laws to protect Social Security numbers but, at present, there is no federal law that would prohibit a covered entity from requesting your Social Security number in order for you to exercise your right of access and/or amendment. Despite some trends away from the use of Social Security numbers as identifiers, many health care providers and insurers still use them as a means of identifying records. If this is the case, you may need to provide your Social Security number in order for the covered entity to locate the record. You should, however, check if your state law provides any greater protections for your Social Security number.

11. Cal. Health & Safety Code §123,111 (West 2002).

12. For the rules on the right to an accounting, see HIPAA Privacy Rule, 45 C.F.R. at §164.528.

13. For the rules on the right to notice of privacy practices, see HIPAA Privacy Rule, 45 C.F.R. at §164.520.

14. For the rules on the right to receive confidential communications, see HIPAA Privacy Rule, 45 C.F.R. at §164.522(b).

15. For the rules on the right request restrictions on uses or disclosures of PHI, see HIPAA Privacy Rule, 45 C.F.R. at § 164.522(b).

16. For the rules on the right to complain, see HIPAA Privacy Rule, 45 C.F.R. at § 160.306.

17. Mearian, L., "Health Net Says 1.5M Medical Records Lost in Data Breach: Connecticut A.G. Calls Six-Month Delay in Reporting Loss Incomprehensible," *Computer World*, November 19, 2009, http://www.computerworld.com/s/article/9141172/Health_Net_says_1.5M_medical_records_lost_in_data_breach (accessed August 21, 2010)

18. See Berry, E., "Health Net settles with Connecticut over data breach: The agreement requires the insurer to adopt new security safeguards and comes at the same time that HHS proposes new data security rules. *American Medical News*, July 21, 2010, http://www.ama-assn.org/amednews/2010/07/26/bisa0726.htm

CHAPTER 3

1. Konrad, W., "Medical Problems Could Include Identity Theft," *New York Times*, June 12, 2009, http://www.nytimes.com/2009/06/13/health/13patient.html?_r=1. (Noting that "… victims may eventually discover erroneous information in their medical files during a doctor or hospital visit. And that may pose a bigger danger than the financial risks. The medical records may now contain vital information like blood type, allergies, prescription drug use, or a history of disease that is just plain wrong. In an emergency, doctors could treat you based on this erroneous information.")

2. Health Insurance Portability and Accountability Act, 42 U.S.C 201 et seq. (42 U.S.C. 1320d-2) (1996).

3. HarrisInteractive.com, Harris Poll #74: Millions Believe Personal Medical Information Has Been Lost or Stolen (2008), http://harrisinteractive.com/harris_poll/index.asp?PID=930 (accessed February 19, 2010).

4. Zetter, K., "New Law Floods California With Medical Data Breach Reports," *Wired*, July 9, 2009, http://www.wired.com/threatlevel/2009/07/health-breaches/#ixzz0fc9ffk6r.

5. HHS, "Breaches Impacting 500 or More Individuals," http://www.hhs.gov/ocr/privacy/hipaa/administrative/breachnotificationrule/postedbreaches.html (accessed March 20, 2010).

6. HIPAA Security Rule, 45 C.F.R. pt. 160, pt. 162, pt. 164 (2003).

7. Id. at §164.306(a)(1).

8. Id. at §164.306(a)(2).

9. Id. at §164.306(a)(3).

10. Id. at §164.304.

11. Id. at §164.308(a)(5)(i).

12. Id. at §164.304.

13. Id.

14. Id. at §164.306(d)(1)(ii)(A).

15. Id. at §164.306(d)(1)(ii)(B).

16. Id. at 45 C.F.R. §164.308.

17. Id. at 45 C.F.R. §164.310.

18. Id. at 45 C.F.R. §164.312.

19. Office for Civil Rights; Delegation of Authority, 74 Fed. Reg 38,630 (August 4, 2009).

20. American Recovery and Reinvestment Act of 2009, Pub. L. No. 111-5, §13402(h)(1).

21. HITECH Breach Notification Rule, 74 Fed. Reg. 42768 (August 24, 2009) (to be codified 45 C.F.R. §164.402(2)(iii)).

22. FTC Health Breach Notification Rule, 74 Fed. Reg. 42,962-42,982 (August 25, 2009) (to be codified 16 C.F.R. pt. 318).

23. Id.

24. Id. at 42976.

25. Id.

26. Breach Notification for Unsecured Protected Health Information, 74 Fed. Reg. 42,740-42,770 (August 24, 2009) (to be codified 45 C.F.R. pt. 160, pt. 164).

27. Wugmeister, M., and Taylor, N. D., "United States: Six States Now Require Social Security Number Protection Policies," December 10, 2008, http://www.mondaq.com/article.asp?articleid=71322.

28. Cal. Civ. Code §1798.29(a) (2002); see *GAO SSN Publication, supra* note 1, at 14. The California law states that, "Any agency that owns or licenses computerized data that includes personal information shall disclose any breach of the security of the system following discovery or notification of the breach in the security of the data to any resident of California whose unencrypted personal information was, or is reasonably believed to have been required by an unauthorized person."

29. N.Y. Gen. Bus. Law. §899-aa.

30. Id. at §899-aa(2).

31. Id. at §899-aa(3).

32. Id. at §899-aa(2).

33. Conn. Gen. Stat. §42-470.

34. Id. at §42-470(b)(1).

35. Id.

36. Id. at §42-470(b)(2)-(4).

37. Id. at §42-470(a).

38. Ariz. Rev. Stat. §44-1373.

39. Id. at §44-1373(A).

40. Id. at §44-1373(D).

41. Id. at §44-1373(E).

42. Id. at §44-1373. Section K of the statute provides that in this section, "individual" means a resident of the state. Ariz. Rev. Stat. §44-1373(K).

43. Minn. Stat. §325E-59(1)(a) (2008).

44. Id.

45. Minn. Stat. §325E-59(1)(a)(1)-(5) (2008).

46. Id. at §325E-59(1)(a)(6) (2008).

47. Id. at §325E-59(1)(a)(7) (2008).

48. Va. Code Ann. §59.1-443.2 (2008).

49. 2008 Conn. Acts 08-167(1)(b).

50. Id.

51. Id. at 08-167(1)(f).

52. Mich. Comp. Laws §445.84 (2004).

53. Id.

54. Id. at §445.84(3) (2004). The Gramm-Leach-Bliley Act provides privacy guidelines and requirements for financial institutions. See Gramm-Leach-Bliley Act, 15 U.S.C. § 6801 to 6809 (1999).

55. Mont. Code Ann. §2-17-552 (2007).

56. Nev. Rev. Stat. §597.970(1).

57. 201 Mass. Code Regs. 17.00-17.05. These regulations implement the provisions of chapter 93H of the General Laws of Massachusetts.

58. Id.

59. 201 Mass. Code Regs. 17.02.

60. Id. at 17.03.

61. Id. at 17.04(3).

62. Id. at 17.04(5).

63. S.B. 6425, 60th Leg., 2008 Reg. Sess. (Wash. 2008).

64. Id. at Sec. 4.

65. S.B. 1022, 94th Leg., Reg. Sess. (Mich. 2008).

66. Id.

67. Id. The new section would have been Subsection (e) to Michigan Compiled Laws §445.71(1).

68. "Healthcare Hacks on the Rise," info security.com, January 26, 2010, http://www.infosecurity-us.com/view/6806/healthcare-hacks-on-the-rise.

69. "Laptop with Patient Info Stolen," *Rocky Mountain News*, November 29, 2006, http://m.rockymountainnews.com/news/2006/Nov/29/laptop-with-patient-info-stolen/.

70. Editorial, "Safeguarding Private Medical Data," *New York Times*, March 26, 2008, at A2, http://www.nytimes.com/2008/03/26/opinion/26wed2.html.

71. Id.

72. Killian, J., "Stolen Laptop has Information on 14,000 Moses Cane Patients, *News & Record*, Apr. 14, 2009, http://www.news-record.com/content/2009/04/13/article/laptop_stolen_contains_information_from_14000_moses_cone_patients.

73. Id.

74. Moscaritolo, A., "Stolen Daytona Beach Hospital Laptop Contained Patient Info," *SC Magazine*, October 23, 2009, http://www.scmagazineus.com/stolen-daytona-beach-hospital-laptop-contained-patient-info/article/156050/

75. Moscaritolo, A., "Laptop Containing UCSF Medical School Patient Information Stolen," *SC Magazine*, Feb. 1, 2010, http://www.scmagazineus.com/laptop-containing-ucsf-medical-school-patient-information-stolen/article/162788/.

76. Id.

77. Konrad, W., "Medical Problems Could Include Identity Theft," *New York Times,* June 12, 2009, http://www.nytimes.com/2009/06/13/health/13patient.html?_r=1.

78. "N.Y. Hospital Employee Admits Stealing, Selling Patient Data," *Campus Safety Magazine,* Aprril 14, 2008, http://www.campussafetymagazine.com/News/?NewsID=1851.

79. Id.

80. Freeman, L., "Florida Health Fraud Case Breaks New Legal Ground," *Naples Daily News,* September 15, 2006, http://www.naplesnews.com/news/2006/sep/15/florida_health_fraud_case_breaks_new_legal_ground/?local_news.

81. Id.

82. In the Matter of Eli Lilly & Co., No. 012 3214, Complaint, http://www.ftc.gov/os/2002/01/lillycmp.pdf.

83. Id. at 1.

84. Id. at 3.

85. Id. at 3–4.

86. Id. at 2–3.

87. Id. at 3.

88. FTC, "Eli Lilly Settles FTC Charges Concerning Security Breach," FTC Release (January 18, 2002), http://www.ftc.gov/opa/2002/01/elililly.htm.

89. In the Matter of Eli Lilly & Co., No. 012 3214, Agreement Containing Consent Order, http://www.supplierportal.lilly.com/SiteCollectionDocuments/FTC_Consent_Order.pdf.

90. Id. at 3–4.

91. Id. at 4.

92. Id.

93. Lee, H. K., "Kaiser Fined $200,000 For Posting Patient Data on Web," *San Francisco Chronicle,* June 21, 2005, http://articles.sfgate.com/2005-06-21/bay-area/17378321_1_kaiser-spokesman-rick-malaspina-patient-data-patient-information.

94. Id.

95. Martinez, B., "Kaiser E-Mail Glitch Highlights Pitfalls of Placing Personal Health-Data Online," *Wall Street Journal,* August 11, 2000, http://faculty.fullerton.edu/lrenold/FA00HUSR470/Kaiser.htm.

96. Id.

97. Id.

98. Piller, C., "Web Mishap: Kids' Psychological Files Posted," *L.A. Times,* November 7, 2001, at A1-1, http://articles.latimes.com/2001/nov/07/news/mn-1140.

99. Id.

100. Ornstein, C., "Hospital to Punish Snooping on Spears: UCLA Moves to Fire at Least 13 For Looking at the Celebrity's Records," *L.A. Times,* March 15, 2008, http://articles.latimes.com/2008/mar/15/local/me-britney15.

101. Institute for Health Care Research and Policy Georgetown University, "Medical Privacy Stories," Health Privacy Project, http://www.drdaniellebabb.com/docs/privacystories814.pdf.

102. Id.

103. Id.

104. Finn, R., "Arthur Ashe, Tennis Star, Is Dead at 49," *New York Times*, February 8, 1993, http://www.nytimes.com/learning/general/onthisday/bday/0710.html?scp=1&sq=Arthur%20Ashe%20hospital&st=cse.

105. Institute for Health Care Research and Policy Georgetown University, *Medical Privacy* Stories, Health Privacy Project, http://www.drdaniellebabb.com/docs/privacystories814.pdf.

106. Id.; State Profile: Nydia M. Velazquez, *USA Today* Online, http://content.usatoday.com/news/politicselections/CandidateProfile.aspx?ci=1535&oi=H (accessed March 26, 2010).

107. Caruso, D., "Prying N.Y. Hospital Workers Suspended," *Washington Post*, September 25, 2006.

108. Id.

109. Id.

110. *Annette Wise v. Thrifty Payless*, 83 Cal. App. 4th 1296.

111. Id.at 1300.

112. Id. at 1299.

113. Id.at 1300.

114. "Institute for Health Care Research and Policy Georgetown University," *Medical Privacy Stories*, Health Privacy Project, http://www.drdaniellebabb.com/docs/privacystories814.pdf.

115. Id.

116. Id.

117. Bernardo, R., "Woman Who Revealed AIDS Info Gets a Year," *Star Bulletin*, June 10, 2009, at A3.

118. Id.

119. Davis, W., "Court: Posting Medical Info On MySpace Violates Privacy," MediaPost, June 28, 2009, http://www.mediapost.com/publications/index.cfm?fa=Articles.showArticle&art_aid=108791.

120. FTC, "CVS Caremark Settles FTC Charges: Failed to Protect Medical and Financial Privacy of Customers and Employees; CVS Pharmacy Also Pays $2.25 Million to Settle Allegations of HIPAA Violations," February 18, 2009, http://www.ftc.gov/opa/2009/02/cvs.shtm.

121. The Federal Trade Commission Act of 1914 (15 U.S.C §§41-58, as amended).

122. Id.

123. Id.

124. U.S. Department of Health and Human Services, "Frequently Asked Questions About the Disposal of Protected Health Information," http://www.hhs.gov/ocr/privacy/hipaa/enforcement/examples/disposalfaqs.pdf (accessed February 28, 2010).

125. Id.

126. Id.

127. Federal Trade Commission, FTC Consumer Network Sentinel Network Databook for January to December 2009, February 2009, http://www.ftc.gov/sentinel/reports/sentinel-annual-reports/sentinel-cy2008.pdf.

128. Macios, A., "Medical Identity Theft: Will the Real John Doe Please Stand Up?" *For the Record*, June 22, 2009, Vol. 21, No. 13 http://www.fortherecordmag.com/archives/062209p10.shtml

129. Mincer, J., "Patient ID Theft Rises," *Wall Street Journal* Online, November 29, 2009, http://online.wsj.com/article/SB125944755514168145.html.

130. Id.

131. Id.

132. "Breach of Privacy Information at Kern Medical Center," TurnTo23.com, November 30, 2009, http://www.turnto23.com/health/21766435/detail.html.

133. Mearian, L., "Health Net Says 1.5M Medical Records Lost in Data Breach: Connecticut A.G. Calls Six-month Delay in Reporting Loss 'Incomprehensible,'" *Computer World*, November 19, 2009, http://www.computerworld.com/s/article/9141172/Health_Net_says_1.5M_medical_records_lost_in_data_breach.

134. Kirchheimer, S., "Scam Alert: Stealing Your Health by Medical Identity Theft," *AARP Bulletin Today*, September 2006, http://bulletin.aarp.org/yourmoney/scamalert/articles/scam_alert__stealing.html.

135. Id.

136. Andrews, M., "Medical Identity Theft Turns Patients Into Victims," *U.S. News and World Report*, February 29, 2008, http://www.usnews.com/health/family-health/articles/2008/02/29/medical-identity-theft-turns-patients-into-victims.html.

137. Id.

138. "Diagnosis: Identity Theft," *BusinessWeek* Online, January 8, 2007, http://www.businessweek.com/magazine/content/07_02/b4016041.htm?chan=top+news_top+news+index_businessweek+exclusives.

139. Id.

140. Konrad, W., "Medical Problems Could Include Identity Theft," *New York Times*, June 12, 2009, http://www.nytimes.com/2009/06/13/health/13patient.html?_r=1.

141. Id.

142. The rules were originally to take effect on November 1, 2008, but were delayed several times—first to May 1, 2009, then to August 1, 2009, then to November 1, 2009, and finally to June 1, 2010. Federal Trade Commission, "FTC Extends Enforcement Deadline for Identity Theft Red Flags Rule," October 10, 2009, http://www.ftc.gov/opa/2009/10/redflags.shtm.

143. Id.

144. The term "creditor" is defined by the Equal Credit Opportunity Act as any person who regularly extends, renews, or continues credit; any person who regularly arranges for the extension, renewal, or continuation of credit; or any assignee of an original creditor who participates in the decision to extend, renew, or continue credit. According to the same act, the term "credit" means the right granted by a creditor to a debtor to defer payment of debt or to incur debts and defer its payment or to

purchase property or services and defer payment thereof. Federal Trade Commission, "New 'Red Flag' Requirements for Financial Institutions and Creditors Will Help Fight Identity Theft," http://www.ftc.gov/bcp/edu/pubs/business/alerts/alt050.shtm (accessed February 28, 2010).

145. FTC Red Flag Rules, 72 Fed. Reg. 63718, 63772 (November 9, 2007) (to be codified at 16 C.F.R. pt. 681).

146. Id.

147. Id.

148. Id. at 63773.

149. *American Medical Association, the American Osteopathic Association and the Medical Society of the District of Columbia v. Federal Trade Commission,* Complaint, http://www.ama-assn.org/ama1/pub/upload/mm/395/red-flags-lawsuit.pdf.

150. "Physicians File Lawsuit on FTC's Red Flags Rule," American Medical Association Online, May 21, 2010, http://www.ama-assn.org/ama/pub/news/news/lawsuit-red-flags-rule.shtml.

151. Id.

152. Id.

153. Id.

154. Id.

155. Robeznieks, A., "Lawsuit Wants to Block Docs From 'Red Flag's' Rule," *Modern Healthcare*, May 26, 2010, http://www.modernhealthcare.com/article/20100526/NEWS/100529941/1153#.

CHAPTER 4

1. HIPAA Privacy Rule, 45 C.F.R. pt. 160, pt. 164 (2000).

2. HIPAA Security Rule, 45 C.F.R. pt. 160, pt. 162, pt. 164 (2003).

3. FamilyHealthGuy, "HIPAA-Potamus," http://blogs.msdn.com/familyhealthguy/archive/2008/05/03/hipaa-potamus.aspx (accessed February 18, 2010).

4. Microsoft's approach to this issue is described in a very interesting position paper, "Microsoft HealthVault and HIPAA," June 2009, http://msdn.microsoft.com/en-us/healthvault/cc507320.aspx (accessed April 9, 2010).

5. On this point, Microsoft's communication stated:

- HIPAA covers health care organizations. Microsoft is not a covered entity by virtue of offering HealthVault. Simply put, HealthVault is not a:
- Health plan because it does not provide insurance.
- Health care clearinghouse because it does not convert health data into or out of standard formats as defined by HIPAA.
- Health care provider because it does not provide health care or services as defined by HIPAA (that is, HealthVault does not provide users with medical or diagnostic advice or health-related products or services).
- Sponsor of Medicare prescription drug cards.

Id.

6. Family Health Guy, "You Put Your Right HIPAA In," http://blogs.msdn.com/ familyhealthguy/archive/2009/06/03/you-put-your-right-hipaa-in.aspx   (accessed April 9, 2010).

7. *FTC v. Toysmart.com, LLC and Toysmart.com, Inc.*, Civil Action No. 00=11341-RGS, Stipulated Consent Agreement and Final Order, http://www.ftc. gov/os/2000/07/toysmartconsent.htm.

8. Federal Trade Commission, "FTC Announces Settlement with Bankrupt Web site, Toysmart.com Regarding Alleged Privacy Policy Violations," FTC Release, July 21, 2000, http://www.ftc.gov/opa/2000/07/toysmart2.shtm.

9. Id.

10. Id.

11. *FTC v. Toysmart.com, LLC and Toysmart.com, Inc.*, Civil Action No. 00=11341-RGS, Stipulated Consent Agreement and Final Order, http://www.ftc. gov/os/2000/07/toysmartconsent.htm.

12. Federal Trade Commission, "Microsoft Settles FTC Charges Alleging False Security and Privacy Promises," FTC Release, August 8, 2002, http://www.ftc.gov/ opa/2002/08/microsoft.shtm.

13. In the Matter of Guess? Inc. and Guess.com, Inc., File No. 022 3260, Complaint, http://www.ftc.gov/opa/2003/06/guess.htm.

14. Id. at 3.

15. Id.

16. Id. at 2.

17. Id. at 4.

18. In the Matter of Guess? Inc. and Guess.com, Inc., File No. 022 3260, Agreement Containing Consent Order, http://www.ftc.gov/opa/2003/06/guess.htm.

19. In the Matter of Petco Animal Supplies, Inc. Complaint, http://www.ftc.gov/ os/caselist/0323221/041108comp0323221.pdf.

20. Id. at 2.

21. Id. at 4.

22. Federal Trade Commission, "Petco Settles FTC Charges. Security Flaws Allowed Hackers to Access Consumers' Credit Card Information" November 17, 2004, http://www.ftc.gov/opa/2004/11/petco.htm.

23. Id.

24. See Federal Trade Commission, Gateway Learning Settles FTC Privacy Charges, Company Rented Customer Information it Pledged to Keep Private In the Matter of Gateway Learning Corp., File No. 042 3047, July 7, 2004, http://www.ftc. gov/opa/2004/07/gateway.htm.

25. Id.

26. Id.

27. Id.

28. Id.

29. Id.

30. Federal Trade Commission, "BJ'S Wholesale Club Settles FTC Charges, Agency Says Lax Security Compromised Thousands of Credit and Debit Cards," FTC No. 0423160, June 16, 2005, http://www.ftc.gov/opa/2005/06/bjswholesale.htm.

31. Id.

32. Id.

33. Id.

34. Id.

35. Under the FTC Breach Rule, a breach is the acquisition of unsecured PHR identifiable health information without the authorization of the individual. FTC Health Breach Notification Rule, 16 C.F.R. §318.2(a) (2009).

36. Federal Trade Commission, "Complying with the FTC's Health Breach Notification Rule," http://www.ftc.gov/bcp/edu/pubs/business/idtheft/bus56.shtm (accessed April 6, 2010).

37. FTC Health Breach Notification Rule, 16 C.F.R. §318.3 (2009).

38. Id. at §318.4 (2009).

39. Id. at §318.5 (2009).

40. Id. at §318.6 (2009).

41. HITECH Breach Notification Rule, 74 Fed. Reg. 42768 (August 24, 2009) (to be codified 45 C.F.R. §164.402(2)(iii)).

42. For example, on the issue of terminated accounts, the privacy policy for Microsoft's HealthVault states: "You can close your account at any time by signing into your HealthVault account and editing your account profile. We wait 90 days before permanently deleting your account information in order to help avoid accidental or malicious removal of your health information." Microsoft Health Vault, "Microsoft HealthVault Account Privacy Statement," https://account.healthvault.com/help.aspx?topicid=PrivacyPolicy (accessed April 9, 2010).

43. Vance A., "If Your Password is 123456 just make it HackMe," *New York Times*, January 20, 2010, http://www.nytimes.com/2010/01/21/technology/21password.html.

CHAPTER 5

1. Patient Protection and Affordable Care Act, Pub. L. No. 111-148, 124 Stat. 119 (2010).

2. Singer, K. "ObamaCare: This Might Hurt, Conntact.com," May 10, 2010, http://www.conntact.com/health/10367-obamacare-this-might-hurt.html; Jerry Geisel, "Health Care Voucher Provision May Inflate Employer Costs," *Business Insurance*, April 19, 2010, http://www.businessinsurance.com/article/20100418/ISSUE01/304189969.

3. "Health Care Reform Will Increase Costs, Reduce Benefits, Towers Watson Surveys Find: Employers and Employees Express Similar Concerns on Health Care Reform," TowersWatson.com, January 27, 2010, http://www.towerswatson.com/press/958 (observing that, "with or without health care reform, employers will continue to look for ways to control rising health care costs and provide high-quality health care for their workers and families.").

4. Americans with Disabilities Act of 1990, 42 U.S.C. 12112(d)(4)(2008).

5. 42 U.S.C. 12112(d).

6. At this stage, the employer may not "conduct a medical examination or make inquiries of a job applicant as to whether such applicant is an individual with a disability or a to the nature or severity of such disability." Id. at §12112(d)(2)(A).

7. Id. at §12112(d)(2)(B).

8. 42 USC §12112(d)(2)(a)(2000).

9. U.S. Equal Employment Opportunity Commission. A Technical Assistance Manual on the Employment Provisions (Title I) of the Americans with Disabilities Act, at ch.5 §§5.5(b)(f) (1992).

10. Id. at Ch. 5 §§5.5(b)(f)

11. 42 U.S.C. §12112(d)(3).

12. Id. §12112(d)(3)(B).

13. 42 USC §12112(d)(4)(A).

14. "U.S. Equal Opportunity Commission, Questions and Answers: Enforcement Guidance on Disability Related Inquiries and Medical Examinations of Employees Under the Americans with Disabilities Act (ADA)," 2000, http://www.eeoc.gov/policy/docs/guidance-inquiries.html [hereinafter "Enforcement Guidance"]

15. Lisa Girion and Ricardo Alonso, "Steep Rise Projected for Health Spending," *L.A. Times*, February 22, 2006, http://articles.latimes.com/2006/feb/22/business/fi-healthcost22.

16. The Kaiser Foundation and Health Research Education Trust, Employee Health Benefits, 2008 Annual Survey, http://ehbs.kff.org/pdf/7790.pdf.

17. Capps, K., and Harkey, J. B., "Harkey, Employee Health and Productivity Programs: The Use of Incentives" (June 2008), http://www.incentone.com/files/2008-surveyresults.pdf.

18. *Id.*

19. Kopicki, A., Van Horn, C., and Zukin, C., "Healthy at Work? Unequal Access to Employer Wellness Programs," "WorkTrends," a report of the John J. Heldrich Center for Workforce Development, Edward J. Bloustein School of Planning and Public Policy, at Rutgers University, http://www.heldrich.rutgers.edu/uploadedFiles/Publications/Heldrich_Center_WT18.pdf.

20. For more information on Scotts, see http://www.thescottsmiraclegrocompany.com/

21. Conlin, M., "Get Healthy? Or Else: Inside One Company's All-Out Attack on Medical Costs," *Business Week,* February 26, 2007, 64.

22. Id.

23. Id.

24. Id.

25. Id.

26. Id.

27. Waldmeir, P., "Quest to Reduce Healthcare Costs Spark Public Debate: A US Law and Garden Company's Decision to Sack a Smoking Worker Could, His Lawyer Warns, be a Harbinger of More Punitive Measures," *Financial Times*, December 30, 2006, 5.

28. *Rodrigues v. Scotts Co.*, No. C.A. 07-10104-GAO, 2008 WL 251971 (D. Mass 2008).

29. Merx, K., "Workers' Unhealthy Habits Could Cost Them," *Detroit Free Press*, May 16, 2005.

30. Peters, J., "Company's Smoking Ban Means Off-Hours, Too," *New York Times*, http://www.nytimes.com/2005/02/08/business/08smoking.html.

31. "Is Smoking a Firing Offense?," The Smokers Club, July 12, 2006, http://www.smokersclubinc.com/modules.php?name=News&file=article&sid=856.

32. "Cleveland Clinic to Include Nicotine Testing in Pre-Employment Physicals as Part of Enhanced Wellness Initiative," *Lab. Bus. Week*, July 15, 2007, 1,050.

33. "Cleveland Clinic Bans Hiring of Smokers," *Columbus Disptach*, June 28, 2007, http://www.dispatch.com/live/content/local_news/stories/2007/06/28/clinic_smokers.html

34. HIPAA Nondiscrimination Rules, 71 Fed. Reg. 75014 (December 13, 2006) (to be codified at 26 C.F.R. pt. 54, 29 C.F.R. pt. 2590, 45 C.F.R. pt. 146). [hereinafter "HIPAA Nondiscrimination Rules"].

35. Genetic Information Nondiscrimination Act of 2009, Pub. L. No. 110-233, 122 Stat. 881 (2008).

36. HIPAA Nondiscrimination Rules, supra note 34 at §2590.702.

37. 29 U.S.C. §1182(a)(1) (2008).

38. HIPAA Nondiscrimination Rules, supra note 34.

39. HIPAA Nondiscrimination Rules, supra note 34 at §2590.702(f).

40. Id. at §2590.702(f)(2).

41. Id. at §2590.702(f)(2)(i).

42. Id. at §2590.702(f)(2)(ii).

43. Id. at 2590.

44. Id. at §2590.702(f)(2)(iii).

45. Id. at §2590.702(f)(2)(iv).

46. According to the wellness regulations, "A plan or issuer may seek verification, such as a statement from an individual's physician, that a health factor makes it unreasonably difficult or medically inadvisable for the individual to satisfy or attempt to satisfy the otherwise applicable standard." HIPAA Nondiscrimination Rules. supra note 34 at §2590.702(f)(2)(iv)(B).

47. Id at §2590.702(f)(3), example 5.

48. Note that this strategy has been informally approved by the U.S. Department of Labor in an interpretation of the proposed wellness rules. In its annual question-and-answer session with the Joint Committee on Employee Benefits of the American Bar Association, the Department of Labor addressed a similar issue, http://www.abanet.org/jceb/2005/qa05dol.pdf (accessed March 7, 2010).

49. HIPAA Nondiscrimination Rules, supra note 34 at§2590.702(f)(2)(v)(A)).

50. Id at §2590.702(f)(2)(v)(B) (2006).

51. Id. at §12112(d)(4)(A).

52. ADA, supra note 2; see also EEOC Enforcement Guidance on Disability-Related Inquiries and Medical Examinations of Employees under the ADA, 8 Fair Empl. Prac. Man. (BNA) 405:7701, http://www.eeoc.gov/policy/docs/guidance-inquiries.html (2000) (hereinafter Enforcement Guidance).

53. Enforcement Guidance, supra note 14.

54. ADA, supra note 2.

55. 29 C.F.R. §1630.14(d) (2000) ("A covered entity may conduct voluntary medical examinations and activities, including voluntary medical histories, which are part of an employee health program available to employees at the work site.").

56. Enforcement Guidance, supra note 14.

57. EEOC Informal Discussion Letter, "ADA: Disability-Related Inquiries and Medical Examinations; Health Risk Assessment," March 6, 2009, http://www.eeoc.gov/eeoc/foia/letters/2009/ada_disability_medexam_healthrisk.html.

58. EEOC Informal Discussion Letter, "ADA: Disability-Related Inquiries and Medical Examinations; Health Risk Assessment," March 6, 2009, http://www.eeoc.gov/eeoc/foia/letters/2009/ada_disability_medexam_healthrisk.html.

59. Id.

60. EEOC Informal Discussion Letter, "ADA: Health Risk Assessments," August 10, 2009, http://www.eeoc.gov/eeoc/foia/letters/2009/ada_health_risk_assessment.html.

61. Id.

62. Id.

63. Genetic Information Nondiscrimination Act of 2009, Pub. L. No. 110-233, 122 Stat. 881 (2008).

64. 45 C.F.R. pt. 144, 146, 148 (2009).

65. HIPAA Nondiscrimination Rules, supra note 34, at §2590.702-1(a)(3).

66. Id. at §2590.702-1(a)(5).

67. Id. at§2590.702-1(d)(1)(ii).

68. 29 U.S.C. §1182 (as amended by GINA) (2008).

69. HIPAA Nondiscrimination Rules supra note 34 at §2590.702-1(d).

70. Id. at §2590.702-1(d)(3).

71. HIPAA Privacy Rule, 45 C.F.R. pt. 160, pt. 164 (2000).

72. 29 C.F.R. §1630.14 (2000).

73. Id.

74. Centers for Disease Control, "Smoking & Tobacco Use, Health Effects of Tobacco Use," http://www.cdc.gov/tobacco/data_statistics/fact_sheets/health_effects/effects_cig_smoking/ (accessed May 17, 2010).

75. "Athlete Study Exposes Flaw of BMI Obesity Measure," FoxNews.com, March 8, 2005, http://www.foxnews.com/story/0,2933,149807,00.html.

76. Rives, A. L., "You're Not the Boss of Me: A Call for Federal Lifestyle Discrimination Legislation," 74 Geo. Wash. L. Rev. 553 at 558 (2006). (Quoting Kim Norris, "His Ultimatum: Quit Smoking or Lose Job," Detroit Free Press, February 15, 2005, 1A).

77. Id.

78. Sandoval, E., and Lucadamo, K., "Whole Foods to Give Greater Employee Discounts to Workers With Lower BMI, Cholesterol," New York Daily News, January 26, 2010, http://www.nydailynews.com/lifestyle/health/2010/01/26/2010-01-26_whole_foods_to_give_greater_employee_discounts_to_workers_with_lower_bmi_cholest.html#ixzz0nfRpqIwJ.

79. Id.

80. Mackey, R., "Depressed Woman Appears Happy on Facebook, Trouble Ensues," New York Times News Blog, November 23, 2009, http://thelede.blogs.

nytimes.com/2009/11/23/depressed-woman-appears-happy-on-facebook-trouble-ensues/?scp=1&sq=nathalie%20blanchard&st=cse.

81. *Mann v. Department of Family and Protective Services,* 2009 WL 2961396 (Tex. App. September 17, 2009)

82. Id.

83. Kwang, K., "Job Hunters Should Avoid Risky Online Behavior," ZDNet Asia, May 7, 2010, http://www.zdnetasia.com/job-hunters-should-avoid-risky-online-behavior-62063098.htm.

CHAPTER 6

1. "$2.3 Trillion Spent on Health Care in 2008: Federal Study Shows Spending Actually Slowed Due to Recession, but That's Still an Average of $7,681 Per Person," CBS News.com, January 5, 2010, http://www.cbsnews.com/stories/2010/01/05/politics/main6057429.shtml.

2. Long, D., "U.S. Pharmaceutical Market Trends: Tremendous Slowdown," IMSHealth.com July, 2009, http://www.imshealth.com/portal/site/imshealth/menu-item.a46c6d4df3db4b3d88f611019418c22a/?vgnextoid=bd34c71e81a32210VgnV CM100000ed152ca2RCRD&vgnextchannel=ad97a7a4fa712210VgnVCM100000 ed152ca2RCRD&vgnextfmt=default.

3. HIPAA Privacy Rule 45 C.F.R. §164.501 (2002).

4. Recall that authorizations were discussed in some detail in Chapter 2. Please refer back to that chapter for additional guidance on authorizations.

5. HIPAA Privacy Rule 45 C.F.R. §164.501 (2002).

6. Id.

7. Health Information Technology for Economic and Clinical Health Act, 123 Stat. at 226 (2009).

8. Id at §13405(a).

9. Id. at §13405(d).

10. Id. at §13405(b)(1)(B) (2009).

11. Id. at §13406.

12. Cal. Civil Code §1798.91 (West 2005).

13. "Workshop on the HIPAA Privacy Rule's De-Identification Standard," http://www.hhs.gov/ocr/privacy/hipaa/understanding/coveredentities/De-identification/deidentificationworkshop2010.html (accessed May 25, 2010).

14. Id.

15. HIPAA Privacy Rule 45 C.F.R. §164.514(b) (2002).

16. Id.

17. Id.

18. Singer, N., "When 2+2 Equals a Privacy Question," *New York Times*, October 17, 2009, http://www.nytimes.com/2009/10/18/business/18stream.html?scp=3&sq=%22de-identified%22&st=cse.

19. Id.

20. Freudheim, M., "And You Thought a Prescription Was Private," *New York Times*, August 8, 2009, http://www.nytimes.com/2009/08/09/business/09privacy. html?sq=de-identified%20health%20data&st=cse&scp=1&pagewanted=all.

21. Id.

22. Id.

23. Id.

24. "Hospital Prescription Records: Study Looks At Re-Identification Risks For Patients," *Science Daily* Online, October 14, 2009, http://www.sciencedaily.com/ releases/2009/10/091014102023.htm.

25. Felch, J., "DNA Profiles Blocked from Public Access," *L.A. Times*, August 29, 2008, A31.

26. "Workshop on the HIPAA Privacy Rule's De-Identification Standard," http:// www.hhs.gov/ocr/privacy/hipaa/understanding/coveredentities/De-identification/ deidentificationworkshop2010.html (accessed May 25, 2010).

27. Freudenheim, *supra* note 20.

28. Singer, *supra* note 18.

29. Vivian, J. C., "Pharmacists Beware: Data Mining Unlawful," USPharmacist. com, June 18, 2009, http://www.uspharmacist.com/content/d/pharmacy_law/c/ 13856/.

30. Freudenheim, *supra* note 20.

31. Singer, *supra* note 18.

32. *IMS Health v. Ayotte*, 550 *F.* 3d 42 at 45, 73-74 (1st Cir. 2008), petition for cert. filed 2009 WL 797587 (U.S. March 27, 2009) (No. 08-1202) (upholding the constitutionality of the New Hampshire Prescription Law).

33. Id. at 45.

34. Id.`

35. Id.

36. Field, A., "Legal Briefing: Will Drugmakers' Prescription Data Mining Be Undermined?" *Daily Finance,* April 3, 2010, http://www.dailyfinance.com/ story/company-news/legal-briefing-will-drugmakers-prescription-data-mining-be-und/19425393/

37. "The Prescription Project, Fact Sheet: Prescription Data Mining," November 19, 2008, http://www.prescriptionproject.org/tools/initiatives_factsheets/files/0004. pdf.

38. Id.

39. N.H. REV. STAT. ANN §318:47-f (2006).

40. Whitney, J., "How Drug Reps Know Which Doctors to Target. Big (Brother) Pharma." *New Republic* Online, August 29, 2006, http://www.reduceddrugprices. org/read.asp?news=389

41. IMS Health, 550 F.3d at 45.

42. Id. at 62-64.

43. Supreme Court Orders, June 29, 2009, http://www.supremecourt.gov/ orders/courtorders/062909zor.pdf.

44. ME REV. STAT. ANN. tit. 22, § 1711 (2007).

45. Vivian, *supra* note 29.

46. *IMS Health v. Mills,* Slip Opinion No. 08-1248, U.S. App (1ˢᵗ Cir Aug.4, 2010), [opinion available at: http://www.ca1.uscourts.gov/cgi-bin/getopn.pl?OPINION=08-1248P.01A

47. Vermont's Prescription Confidentiality Law, VT. STAT. ANN. tit. 18, §4631 (2009).

48. *IMS Health v. Sorrell,* 631 F. Supp. 2d 434 (2009).

49. Vivian, *supra* note 29.

50. Id.

51. You can, for example, add your name to name-deletion lists used nationwide by marketers. To find out how, visit http://www.dmachoice.org. You can also add your name to the National Do-Not-Call Registry at http://www.fcc.gov/cgb/donotcall.

CHAPTER 7

1. Waller, A., "Health Care Issues in Health Care Reform," 16 *Whittier L. Rev.* 15, 44 (1995).

2. One notable exception to this basic rule can be found in how the HIPAA Privacy Rule treats psychotherapy notes differently from other types of PHI. See HIPAA Privacy Rule, 45 C.F.R. §164.501 (2000). The issue of psychotherapists' notes will be discussed in more detail in subsequent sections.

3. HIPAA Privacy Rule, 45 C.F.R. §§164.502(b); 164.508 (2000).

4. Id. at §164.514(d)(2).

5. Id. at §164.510.

6. Id. at §164.512.

7. Id. at 45 C.F.R. §508(c).

8. The Drug Abuse Prevention, Treatment, and Rehabilitation Act, 21 U.S.C. 1175, was transferred to section 527 of the Public Health Service Act, codified at 42 U.S.C. 290ee-3 and then later transferred to §290dd-2. The Comprehensive Alcohol Abuse and Alcoholism Prevention, Treatment, and Rehabilitation Act of 1970 (42 U.S.C. 4582) was amended and transferred to section 523 of the Public Health Service Act, codified at 42 U.S.C. 290dd-3 and eventually omitted, presumably because confidentiality for alcohol treatment was eventually bundled with confidentiality for substance use treatment.

9. Confidentiality of Alcohol and Drug Abuse Patient Records, 42 C.F.R. pt. 2.

10. Id. at 42 C.F.R. §2.2 (b).

11. Id. at 42 C.F.R. §2.11.

12. Id.

13. Id. at 42 C.F.R. §2.3(b)(3), 2.4.

14. Id. at §2.12(d).

15. Id. at 42 C.F.R. §2.11.

16. Id.

17. Id.

18. Id. at 42 C.F.R. §2.13(a).

19. Id.

20. Id. at 42 C.F.R. 2.6.

21. Id. at 42 C.F.R. §2.12(b).

22. Id at. 42 C.F.R. §2.12(c).

23. Id. at 42 C.F.R. §2.32.

24. Id. at 42 C.F.R. §2.20.

25. Family Education Rights and Privacy Act of 1974, 20 U.S.C.§1232g (2002).

26. Id. at §1232g(d).

27. Id. at §1232(g)(4)(A).

28. 65 Fed. Reg. 82,462, 82,621 (to be codified 45 C.F.R. pt. 160, 164) (2000).

29. 42 C.F.R. §§431.300-431.307 (1998).

30. *Mental Health: A Report of the Surgeon General,* Chapter 7, Current State of Confidentiality Law, http://www.surgeongeneral.gov/library/mentalhealth/chapter7/sec3.html (accessed February 20, 2010).

31. Id.

32. N.Y. Mental Hygiene Law §33 (2010).

33. Id. at §33.13(c)(1).

34. HIPAA Privacy Rule, 45 C.F.R. §§164.502(a)(1) (2000).

35. N.Y. Mental Hygiene Law §33.13(c)(7) (2010).

36. Doughty, R., "The Confidentiality of HIV-Related Information: Responding to the Resurgence of Aggressive Public Health Intervention in the AIDS Epidemic," 82 *Cal. L. Rev.* 111 (1994).

37. *Estate of Behringer v. Medical Center at Princeton,* 249 N.J. Super. 597, 641 (Law Div. 1991).

38. Department of Health and Human Services Project, Health Information Privacy Protections Under Federal and State Law, ABA Health Law Section, October 23, 2006, http://www.allhealth.org/briefingmaterials/hhs-privacy-1103.pdf.

39. Id.

40. N.Y. Pub. Health Law §2781(1).

41. Id.

42. Id. at §2782.

43. Id. at §2783.

44. S.C. Code Ann. §44-29-135(e) (2008) (requiring the DHEC to notify the superintendent and school nurse at the student's school if a student tests positive for human immunodeficiency virus [HIV] or acquired immune deficiency syndrome [AIDS]).

45. Jones, R. C., *Living With HIV/AIDS: Students Tell Their Stories of Stigma, Courage, and Resillience* 22–32 (2006), http://www.nsba.org/MainMenu/School-Health/SelectedNSBAPublications/HIVAIDS.aspx.

46. Centers for Disease Control and Prevention, "Estimates of New HIV Infections in the United States 6" (August 2008), http://www.cdc.gov/hiv/topics/surveillance/resources/factsheets/incidence.htm promotes testing to increase awareness and prevent the transmission of HIV).

47. Ping Tsao, C. I., Tummala A., and Weiss Roberts, L., "Editorial: Stigma in Mental Health Care," *Acad Psychiatry* 32:70–72 (March–April 2008).

48. Utah Code Ann. §§58-61-602; 58-60-509; 58-60-114.

49. Id.

50. Pa. Stat. Ann. tit. 35, §521.4.

51. 28 Pa. Code §§27.21a; 27.22; 27.23.

52. Pa. Stat. Ann. tit. 35, §521.15.

53. Id.

54. Pa. Stat. Ann. tit. 35, §521.20.

55. Privacy Act of 1974, 5 U.S.C. §552a (2006).

56. *Cooper v. Federal Aviation Administration*, 3:07-cv-01383-VRW (N.D.C.A. August 22, 2009), http://www.scribd.com/doc/5573405/CooperVFAA-08-22-08.

57. *Estate of Behringer v. Medical Center at Princeton*, 249 N.J. Super. 597, 641 (Law Div. 1991).

58. Id. at 641.

59. *Roe v. Social Security Administration* (03-CIV-3812; settled 2004), "The Legal Action Centers Leading Cases," http://www.lac.org/doc_library/lac/publications/leading_cases.pdf (accessed May 24, 2010).

60. Id.

61. *Randi A. J. v. Long Island Surgi-Center*, 46 A.D.3d 74 (2d Dep't. 2007).

62. Id. at 80.

63. Id.

64. Id. at 75.

65. Id, at 75–76.

66. Id. at 83.

CHAPTER 8

1. Regarding Canada, see, e.g., Merrill, M., "Virus Blamed for EHR Breach in Canada," *HealthCare IT News*, July 9 2009, http://www.healthcareitnews/virus-blamed-her-breach-Canada; "N.W.T. Medical Records Faxed to CBC," CBC, http://www.cbc.ca/canada/north/story/2010/05/11/nwt-medical-records-fax.html. Regarding Australia, see Laird, C., "Medicare Privacy Breaches 'Only the Beginning,'" ABC News (Australia), March 2, 2010, http://www.anc.net.au/news/stories/2010/03/02/2834702.htm. Regarding the United Kingdom, see Savage, M., "NHS 'Loses' Thousands of Medical Records," *The Independent*, May 25, 2009, http://www.independent.co.uk/news/uk/politics/nhs-loses-thousands-of-medical-records-1690398.html.

2. On the debate in the UK, see: http://www.yourprivacy.co.uk/yourmedicalrecords.html (accessed May 23, 2010). On the debate in Australia, see "Your Privacy at Risk—Frequently Asked Questions," Australian Medical Associates, http://www.ama.au/node/4629

3. The Personal Information Protection and Electronic Documents Act, 2000 S.C., ch. 5 (Can.).

4. Id. §3.

5. Office of the Privacy Commissioner of Canada, "Your Privacy Responsibilities: Canada's Personal Information Protection and Electronic Documents Act," http://www.priv.gc.ca/information/guide_e.pdf (accessed May 17, 2010).

6. Id.

7. Office of the Privacy Commissioner of Canada, "Legal Information Related to PIPEDA: Interpretations (Personal Information)," http://www.priv.gc.ca/leg_c/interpretations_02_e.cfm (accessed May 17, 2010).

8. Id.

9. The Personal Information Protection and Electronic Documents Act, 2000 S.C., ch. 5 §2.

10. Office of the Privacy Commissioner of Canada, "Legal Information Related to PIPEDA: Implementation Schedule," http://www.priv.gc.ca/legislation/02_06_02a_e.cfm (accessed May 18, 2010).

11. Id.

12. Id.

13. The Personal Information Protection and Electronic Documents Act, 2000 S.C., ch. 5 §2(1).

14. The code is available through CSA Standards, http://www.csa.ca/cm/ca/en/privacy-code.

15. The Personal Information Protection and Electronic Documents Act, 2000 S.C., ch. 5 §7.

16. Id.

17. Id.

18. Office of the Privacy Commissioner of Canada, "Summaries of Cases Settled During the Course of the Investigation under the Personal Information Protection and Electronic Documents Act," http://www.privcom.gc.ca/ser/index_01_e.asp (accessed April 14, 2010).

19. Office of the Privacy Commissioner of Canada, "Summary of an Early Resolution Case Under the Personal Information Protection and Electronic Documents Act," http://www.privcom.gc.ca/ser/index_02_e.asp (accessed April 14, 2010).

20. Privacy Act 1988 (Australia), http://www.comlaw.gov.au/ComLaw/Legislation/ActCompilation1.nsf/framelodgmentattachments/80B97C0EECC31CA4CA2576BF007FBEBD (accessed April 14, 2010).

21. Office of the Privacy Commissioner (Australia), "Privacy in the Private Health Sector," November 9, 2001, http://www.privacy.gov.au/materials/types/guidelines/view/6517 (accessed April 14, 2010).

22. Id. app. 2.

23. Id. pt. A.3.2.

24. Id. pt. A.3.5.

25. Id. pt. A.3.4.

26. Australian Law Reform Commission, "ALRC Report 108: For Your Information: Australian Privacy Law and Practice," http://www.austlii.edu.au/au/other/alrc/publications/reports/108/#Contents.

27. Id.

28. Australian Law Reform Commission, "Media Release: Government gives giant 'tick' to ALRC privacy recommendations," October 14, 2009, http://www.alrc.gov.au/media/2009/mr1410.html.

29. Directive 1995/46, 1995 O.J. (L 281) 31 (EC).

30. Id. at art. 2(a).

31. Id. at art. 4, which provides:

    1. Each Member State shall apply the national provisions it adopts pursuant to this Directive to the processing of personal data where:

        a. the processing is carried out in the context of the activities of an establishment of the controller on the territory of the Member State; when the same controller is established on the territory of several Member States, he must take the necessary measures to ensure that each of these establishments complies with the obligations laid down by the national law applicable;

b. the controller is not established on the Member State's territory, but in a place where its national law applies by virtue of international public law;

c. the controller is not established on Community territory and, for purposes of processing personal data makes use of equipment, automated or otherwise, situated in the territory of the said Member State, unless such equipment is used only for purposes of transit through the territory of the Community.

Id.

32. Id. at art. 7(a).

33. Id. at art. 8(1).

34. Id. at art. 8(2).

35. Id. at art. 28 (requiring each member state to "provide that one or more public authorities are responsible for the application within its territory of the provisions adopted by the Member States pursuant to this directive.").

36. Id. at art. 19(1).

37. Id. at art. 12(a).

38. Id.

39. Id. at art. 17(1).

40. Id. at art. 17(2).

41. B.O.E. 1999, 151, art. 4(2).

42. Directive, *supra* note 20, at art. 17(2).

43. Id.

44. Id. at art. 25.

45. Id.

46. "Discussion Document: First Orientations on Transfers of Personal Data to Third Countries—Possible Ways Forward in Assessing Adequacy," June 26,1997, WP 4, http://ec.europa.eu/justice_home/fsj/privacy/docs/wpdocs/1997/wp4_en.pdf.

47. "Working Document on the Processing of Personal Data Relating to Health in Electronic Health Records," http://ec.europa.eu/justice_home/fsj/privacy/docs/wpdocs/2007/wp131_en.pdf (accessed May 23, 2010).

48. Id.

49. "Europe Aims for Borderless Electronic Health Records," eHealthEurope, July 2, 2008, http://www.ehealtheurope.net/News/3911/europe_aims_for_borderless_electronic_health_records.

CONCLUSION

1. American Medical Association, Code of Medical Ethics, http://www.ama-assn.org/ama/pub/physician-resources/medical-ethics/code-medical-ethics.shtml at 5.05:

The information disclosed to a physician by a patient should be held in confidence. The patient should feel free to make a full disclosure of information to the physician in order that the physician may most effectively provide needed services. The patient should be able to make this disclosure with the knowledge that the physician will respect the confidential nature of the communication. The physician should not reveal confidential information without the express consent of the patient, subject to certain exceptions that are ethically justified because of overriding considerations.

When a patient threatens to inflict serious physical harm to another person or to him or herself and there is a reasonable probability that the patient may carry out the threat, the physician should take reasonable precautions for the protection of the intended victim, which may include notification of law enforcement authorities.

When the disclosure of confidential information is required by law or court order, physicians generally should notify the patient. Physicians should disclose the minimal information required by law, advocate for the protection of confidential information and, if appropriate, seek a change in the law.

Opinion 5.05, which sets forth general duties of confidentiality, is included as an illustrative example. Additional provisions of the AMA's Code of Medical Ethics also address the physician's duty to respect the privacy of patients and maintain patient confidentiality. Also interesting in this regard is Opinion 5.059, which provides:

In the context of health care, emphasis has been given to confidentiality, which is defined as information told in confidence or imparted in secret. However, physicians also should be mindful of patient privacy, which encompasses information that is concealed from others outside of the patient-physician relationship.

Physicians must seek to protect patient privacy in all of its forms, including (1) physical, which focuses on individuals and their personal spaces, (2) informational, which involves specific personal data, (3) decisional, which focuses on personal choices, and (4) associational, which refers to family or other intimate relations. Such respect for patient privacy is a fundamental expression of patient autonomy and is a prerequisite to building the trust that is at the core of the patient-physician relationship.

Privacy is not absolute, and must be balanced with the need for the efficient provision of medical care and the availability of resources. Physicians should be aware of and respect the special concerns of their patients regarding privacy. Patients should be informed of any significant infringement on their privacy of which they may otherwise be unaware.

GLOSSARY

1. 45 CFR §160.103.

Select Bibliography

CASE LAW

Annette Wise v. Thrifty Payless, 83 Cal. App. 4th 1296 (2000).

Cooper v. Federal Aviation Administration, 3:07-cv-01383-VRW (N.D.C.A. August 22, 2009), http://www.scribd.com/doc/5573405/CooperVFAA-08-22-08.

Estate of Behringer v. Medical Center at Princeton, 249 N.J. Super. 597, 641 (Law Div. 1991).

FTC v. Toysmart.com, LLC and Toysmart.com, Inc., Civil Action No. 00=11341-RGS, Stipulated Consent Agreement and Final Order, http://www.ftc.gov/os/2000/07/toysmartconsent.htm.

IMS Health v. Ayotte, 550 F. 3d 42 at 45, 73-74 (1st Cir. 2008), petition for cert. filed, 2009 WL 797587 (U.S. March 27, 2009) (No. 08-1202) (upholding the constitutionality of the New Hampshire Prescription Law).

IMS Health v. Sorrell, 631 F. Supp. 2d 434 (2nd Cir. 2009).

In the Matter of Eli Lilly & Co., No. 012 3214, Agreement Containing Consent Order, http://www.supplierportal.lilly.com/SiteCollectionDocuments/FTC_Consent_Order.pdf.

In the Matter of Eli Lilly & Co., No. 012 3214, Complaint, http://www.ftc.gov/os/2002/01/lillycmp.pdf.

In the Matter of Guess? Inc. and Guess.com, Inc., File No. 022 3260, Agreement Containing Consent Order http://www.ftc.gov/os/2003/08/guessdo.pdf

In the Matter of Guess? Inc. and Guess.com, Inc., File No. 022 3260, Complaint, http://www.ftc.gov/os/2003/08/guesscomp.pdf

In the Matter of Petco Animal Supplies, Inc. Complaint, http://www.ftc.gov/os/caselist/0323221/041108comp0323221.pdf.

Olmstead v. United States, 277 U.S. 438, 478 (1928) (Brandeis, J., dissenting).

Randi A.J. v. Long Island Surgi-Center, 46 A.D.3d 74 (2nd Dep't. 2007).

FEDERAL AND INTERNATIONAL REGULATIONS

Americans with Disabilities Act of 1990, 42 U.S.C 12101(2008).

American Recovery and Reinvestment Act of 2009, Pub. L. No. 111-5, §13402(h)(1) (2009).

Breach Notification for Unsecured Protected Health Information, 74 Fed. Reg. 42,740-42,770 (August 24, 2009) (to be codified 45 C.F.R. pt. 160, pt. 164).

Confidentiality of Alcohol and Drug Abuse Patient Records, 42 C.F.R. pt. 2 (2002).

Council Directive 1995/46, 1995 O.J. (L 281) 31 (EC).

EEOC Enforcement Guidance on Disability-Related Inquiries and Medical Examinations of Employees under the ADA, 8 Fair Empl. Prac. Man. (BNA) 405:7701 http://www.eeoc.gov/policy/docs/guidance-inquiries.html (2000).

Family Education Rights and Privacy Act of 1974, 20 U.S.C.§1232g (2002).

FTC Health Breach Notification Rule, 74 Fed. Reg. 42,962-42,982 (August 25, 2009) (to be codified 16 C.F.R. pt. 318).

FTC Red Flag Rules, 72 Fed. Reg. 63718, 63772 (November 9, 2007) (to be codified at 16 C.F.R. pt. 681).

Genetic Information Nondiscrimination Act of 2009, Pub. L. No. 110-233, 122 Stat. 881 (2008).

Gramm-Leach-Bliley Act, 15 U.S.C. § 6801-09 (1999).

Health Information Technology for Economic and Clinical Health Act, 123 Stat. at 226 (2009).

Health Insurance Portability and Accounting Act of 1996, Pub. L. No. 104-191, 110 Stat. 1936 (codified as amended in scattered sections of 42 U.S.C.).

HIPAA Nondiscrimination Rules, 71 Fed. Reg. 75014 (December 13, 2006) (to be codified at 26 C.F.R. pt. 54, 29 C.F.R. pt. 2590, 45 C.F.R. pt. 146).

HIPAA Privacy Rule, 45 C.F.R. pt. 160, pt. 164 (2000). (

HIPAA Security Rule, 45 C.F.R. pt. 160, pt. 162, pt. 164 (2003).

HITECH Breach Notification Rule, 74 Fed. Reg. 42768 (August 24, 2009) (to be codified 45 C.F.R. §164.402(2)(iii)).

Office for Civil Rights; Delegation of Authority, 74 Fed. Reg. 38,630 (August 4, 2009).

Office of Tech. Assessment, Protecting Privacy in Computerized Medical Information, No. 576 (1993).

Office of the Inspector Gen., Dep't of Health and Human Serv., A-04-07-05064, Nationwide Review of the Centers for Medicare & Medicaid Services Health Insurance Portability and Accountability Act of 1996 Oversight (2008).

Patient Protection and Affordable Care Act, H.R. 3590, 111th Cong. §1201 (2009).

Patient Protection and Affordable Care Act, Pub. L. No. 111-148, 124 Stat. 119 (2010).

Personal Information Protection and Electronic Documents Act, 2000 S.C., Ch. 5 (Can.).

Privacy Act of 1974, 5 U.S.C. §552a (2006).

Universal Declaration of Human Rights, G.A. Res. 217A, at 73, U.N. GAOR, 3d Sess., 1st plen. mtg., U.N. Doc. A/810 (December 10, 1948).

STATE LAWS

28 Pa. Code §§27.21a; 27.22; 27.23.

201 Mass. Code Regs. 17.00-17.05

2008 Conn. Acts 08-167(1)

Ariz. Rev. Stat. §44-1373.

Cal. Civ. Code §1798.29(a) (2002)

Conn. Gen. Stat. §42-470.

N.H. Rev. Stat. Ann §318:47-f (2006).

N.Y. Gen. Bus. Law. §899-aa.

N.Y. Mental Hygiene Law(2010).

N.Y. Pub. Health Law(2010).

ME Rev. Stat. Ann. Tit. 22, §1711 (2007).

Mich. Comp. Laws §445.84 (2004).

Minn. Stat. §325E-59(1)(a) (2008).

Mont. Code Ann. §2-17-552 (2007).

Nev. Rev. Stat. §597.970(1).

Pa. Stat. Ann. tit. 35, §521.

S.C. Code Ann. §44-29-135(e) (2008).

Utah Code Ann. §§58-61-602; 58-60-509; 58-60-114.

Va. Code Ann. §59.1-443.2 (2008).

Vermont's Prescription Confidentiality Law, VT. Stat. Ann. tit. 18, §4631 (2009).

LAW REVIEW AND JOURNAL ARTICLES

Adele Waller, "Health Care Issues in Health Care Reform," 16 *Whittier L. Rev.* 15, 44 (1995).

Andis Robeznieks, "Lawsuit Wants to Block Docs From 'Red Flags Rule," *Modern Healthcare*, May 26, 2010, http://www.modernhealthcare.com/article/20100526/NEWS/100529941/1153#.

Ann L. Rives, "You're Not the Boss of Me: A Call for Federal Lifestyle Discrimination" Legislation, 74 *Geo. Wash. L. Rev.* 553 (2006).

Carol I. Ping Tsao, Aruna Tummala, and Laura Weiss Roberts, "Editorial: Stigma in Mental Health Care," *Acad Psychiatry* 32:70–72 (March–April 2008).

Gregory Katz and Stuart O. Schweitzer, "Implications of Genetic Testing for Health Policy," 10 *Yale J. Health Pol'y L. & Ethics* 90, 94 (2010).

Karleen J. Green, "The Benefits of Changing Times: Health Plan Compliance in 2010," 57 *Fed. Law* 36, 38 (2010).

Kenneth M. Siegel, Comment, "Protecting the Most Valuable Corporate Asset: Electronic Data, Identity Theft, Personal Information and the Role of Data Security in the Information Age," 111 *Penn St. L. Rev.* 779, 819 (2007).

Nicolas P. Terry and Leslie P. Francis, "Ensuring the Privacy and Confidentiality of Electronic Health Records," 2007 *U. Ill. L. Rev* 681; see also Adam D. Moore, "Intangible Property: Privacy, Power and Information Control," 35 *Am. Philosophical Q.* 365 (1998).

Roger Doughty, "The Confidentiality of HIV-Related Information: Responding to the Resurgence of Aggressive Public Health Intervention in the AIDS Epidemic," 82 *Cal. L. Rev.* 111 (1994).

Samuel D. Warren and Louis D. Bradeis, "The Right to Privacy," 4 *Harv. L. Rev.* 193, 193 (1890).

Symposium, "Personal Privacy and Common Goods: A Framework for Balancing Under the National Health Information Privacy Rule," 86 *Minn. L. Rev.* 1439 (2002).

Symposium, "Privacy As Contextual Integrity," 79 *Wash. L. Rev.* 119 (2004).

NEWSPAPER AND MAGAZINE ARTICLES

"Cleveland Clinic to Include Nicotine Testing in Pre-Employment Physicals as Part of Enhanced Wellness Initiative," *Lab. Business Week*, July 15, 2007, 1050.

David Caruso, "Prying N.Y. Hospital Workers Suspended," *Washington Post*, Sept. 25, 2006.

Jason Felch, "DNA Profiles Blocked from Public Access," *L.A. Times*, Aug 29 2008, A31.

Kim Norris, "His Ultimatum: Quit Smoking or Lose Job," *Detroit Free Press*, February 15, 2005, 1A.

WEB RESOURCES

Allison Kopicki, Carl Van Horn, and Cliff Zukin, "Healthy at Work? Unequal Access to Employer Wellness Programs," *WorkTrends*, a report of the John J. Heldrich Center for Workforce Development, Edward J. Bloustein School of Planning and Public Policy, Rutgers University, http://www.heldrich.rutgers.edu/uploadedFiles/Publications/Heldrich_Center_WT18.pdf.

Angela Moscaritolo, "Laptop Containing UCSF Medical School Patient Information Stolen," *SC Magazine*, February 1, 2010, http://www.scmagazineus.com/laptop-containing-ucsf-medical-school-patient-information-stolen/article/162788/.

Annual question-and-answer session with the Joint Committee on Employee Benefits of the American Bar Association; the Department of Labor addressed a similar issue, http://www.abanet.org/jceb/2005/qa05dol.pdf (accessed March 7, 2010).

Ashley Vance, "If Your Password is 123456 Just Make it HackMe," *New York Times*, January 20, 2010, http://www.nytimes.com/2010/01/21/technology/21password.html.

"Athlete Study Exposes Flaw of BMI Obesity Measure," Fox News.com March 8, 2005, http://www.foxnews.com/story/0,2933,149807,00.html

Barbara Martinez, "Kaiser E-Mail Glitch Highlights Pitfalls of Placing Personal-Health Data Online," *Wall Street Journal*, August 11, 2000, http://faculty.fullerton.edu/lrenold/FA00HUSR470/Kaiser.htm.

"Breach of Privacy Information at Kern Medical Center," TurnTo23.com, November 30, 2009, http://www.turnto23.com/health/21766435/detail.html.

California Health Care Foundation, "Medical Privacy and Confidentiality Survey (1999)," http://www.chcf.org/topics/view.cfm?itemID=12500.

California Health Care Foundation, "National Consumer Health Privacy Survey (2005)," http://www.chcf.org/topics/view.cfm?itemID=115694.

Centers for Disease Control, "Smoking & Tobacco Use, Health Effects of Tobacco Use" (accessed May 17, 2010), http://www.cdc.gov/tobacco/data_statistics/fact_sheets/health_effects/effects_cig_smoking/.

Centers for Disease Control and Prevention, "Estimates of New HIV Infections in the United States 6," (August 2008), http://www.cdc.gov/hiv/topics/surveillance/ resources/factsheets/incidence/pdf promoting testing to increase awareness and prevent the transmission of HIV).

Centers for Medicare and Medicaid Services, http://www.cms.hhs.gov/clia.

Charles Ornstein, "Hospital to Punish Snooping on Spears: UCLA Moves to Fire at Least 13 For Looking at the Celebrity's Records," *L.A. Times*, March 15, 2008, http://articles.latimes.com/2008/mar/15/local/me-britney15.

Charles Piller, "Web Mishap: Kids' Psychological Files Posted," *L.A. Times*, November 7, 2001, A1-1, http://articles.latimes.com/2001/nov/07/news/mn-1140.

"Cleveland Clinic Bans Hiring of Smokers," *Columbus Dispatch*, June 28, 2007, http://www.dispatch.com/live/content/local_news/stories/2007/06/28/clinic_ smokers.html.

"Cleveland Clinic to Include Nicotine Testing in Pre-Employment Physicals as Part of Enhanced Wellness Initiative," *Lab. Business Week*, July 15, 2007, at 1050, http:// www.prnewswire.com/news-releases/cleveland-clinic-to-include-nicotine-testing- in-pre-employment-physicals-as-part-of-enhanced-wellness-initiative-58540132. html.

The Council of State Governors, "Trends in State Health Legislation: STD, HIV/ AIDS, and Teen Pregnancy Prevention January 1 to June 30, 2009," August 26, 2009, http://www.healthystates.csg.org/NR/rdonlyres/3C358B5B-93E7-4AB9- 825E-3BF17163D675/0/Aug2009CSGMidYearReport.pdf.

Department of Health, Education and Welfare (now Department of Health and Human Services), "Records, Computers and the Rights of Citizens: Report of the Secretary's Advisory Committee on Automated Personal Data Systems," http:// aspe.hhs.gov/datacncl/1973privacy/c3.htm.

"Diagnosis: Identity Theft," *Business Week* Online, January 8, 2007, http://www. businessweek.com/magazine/content/07_02/b4016041.htm?chan=top+news_top +news+index_businessweek+exclusives.

Edgar Sandoval and Kathleen Lucadamo, "Whole Foods to Give Greater Employee Discounts To Workers With Lower BMI, Cholesterol," *New York Daily News*, January 26, 2010, http://www.nydailynews.com/lifestyle/health/2010/01/26/2010- 01-26_whole_foods_to_give_greater_employee_discounts_to_workers_with_ lower_bmi_cholest.html#ixzz0nfRpqIwJ.

Editorial, "Safeguarding Private Medical Data," *New York Times*, March 26, 2008, A2, http://www.nytimes.com/2008/03/26/opinion/26wed2.html.

EEOC Informal Discussion Letter, "ADA: Disability-Related Inquiries and Medical Examinations; Health Risk Assessment," March 6, 2009, http://www.eeoc.gov/ eeoc/foia/letters/2009/ada_disability_medexam_healthrisk.html.

EEOC Informal Discussion Letter, "ADA: Health Risk Assessments," August 10, 2009, http://www.eeoc.gov/eeoc/foia/letters/2009/ada_health_risk_assessment.html.

Elizabeth Armstrong Moore, "E-prescriptions More Reliable Than Handwritten Ones," CNET News, February 26, 2010, http://news.cnet.com/8301-27083 _3-10460672-247.html.

"Europe Aims for Borderless Electronic Health Records," eHealthEurope, July 2, 2008, http://www.ehealtheurope.net/News/3911/europe_aims_for_borderless _electronic_health_records.

Family Health Guy, "HIPAA-Potamus," http://blogs.msdn.com/familyhealthguy/ archive/2008/05/03/hipaa-potamus.aspx (accessed February 18, 2010).

Family Health Guy, "You Put Your Right HIPAA In," http://blogs.msdn.com/ familyhealthguy/archive/2009/06/03/you-put-your-right-hipaa-in.aspx (accessed April 9, 2010).

Federal Trade Commission, "BJ's Wholesale Club Settles FTC Charges, Agency Says Lax Security Compromised Thousands of Credit and Debit Cards," FTC No. 0423160 (June 16, 2005), http://www.ftc.gov/opa/2005/06/bjswholesale.htm.

Federal Trade Commission, "CVS Caremark Settles FTC Charges: Failed to Protect Medical and Financial Privacy of Customers and Employees; CVS Pharmacy Also Pays $2.25 Million to Settle Allegations of HIPAA Violations," FTC Release, February 18, 2009, http://www.ftc.gov/opa/2009/02/cvs.shtm.

Federal Trade Commission, "Eli Lilly Settles FTC Charges Concerning Security Breach," FTC Release, January 18, 2002, http://www.ftc.gov/opa/2002/01/elililly.htm.

Federal Trade Commission, "FTC Announces Settlement with Bankrupt Website, Toysmart.com Regarding Alleged Privacy Policy Violations," FTC Release, July 21, 2000, http://www.ftc.gov/opa/2000/07/toysmart2.shtm.

Federal Trade Commission, "FTC Consumer Network Sentinel Network Databook for January to December 2009," February 2009, http://www.ftc.gov/sentinel/ reports/sentinel-annual-reports/sentinel-cy2008.pdf.

Federal Trade Commission, "FTC Testifies on Data Security, Peer-to-Peer File Sharing," May 5, 2009, http://www.ftc.gov/opa/2009/05/peer2peer.shtm.

Federal Trade Commission, "Gateway Learning Settles FTC Privacy Charges: Company Rented Customer Information it Pledged to Keep Private In the Matter of Gateway Learning Corp.," July 7, 2004, http://www.ftc.gov/opa/2004/07/gateway.htm.

Federal Trade Commission, "New 'Red Flag' Requirements for Financial Institutions and Creditors Will Help Fight Identity Theft," http://www.ftc.gov/bcp/edu/pubs/ business/alerts/alt050.shtm (accessed February 28, 2010).

Federal Trade Commission, "Petco Settles FTC Charges. Security Flaws Allowed Hackers to Access Consumers' Credit Card Information," November 17, 2004, http://www.ftc.gov/opa/2004/11/petco.htm.

Fred Schulte, "Stimulus Fuels Gold Rush For Electronic Health Systems," *Huffington Post*, November 9, 2009, http://www.huffingtonpost.com/2009/11/05/stimulus- fuels-gold-rush_n_347311.html

Fred Schulte and Emma Schwartz, "Experts: Move To Electronic Medical Records Needs Oversight," *Huffington Post*, February 25, 2010, http://www.huffington- post.com/2010/ 02/25/experts-move-to-electroni_n_477546.html.

Harris Poll #74, Harris Interactive, "Millions Believe Personal Medical Information Has Been Lost or Stolen: Issue a Roadblock to Acceptance of Electronic Health Record Systems," July 15, 2008, http://www.harrisinteractive.com/harris_poll/ index.asp?PID=930.

"Health Care Reform Will Increase Costs, Reduce Benefits, Towers Watson Surveys Find: Employers and Employees Express Similar Concerns on Health Care

Reform," TowersWatson.com, January 27, 2010, http://www.towerswatson.com/press/958.

Henry K. Lee, "Kaiser Fined $200,000 For Posting Patient Data on Web," *San Francisco Chronicle*, June 21, 2005, http://articles.sfgate.com/2005-06-21/bay-area/17378321_1_kaiser-spokesman-rick-malaspina-patient-data-patient-information.

"Hospital Prescription Records: Study Looks At Re-Identification Risks For Patients," Science Daily Online, October 14, 2009, http://www.sciencedaily.com/releases/2009/10/091014102023.htm.

Institute for Health Care Research and Policy Georgetown University, "Medical Privacy Stories," Health Privacy Project, http://www.drdaniellebabb.com/docs/privacystories814.pdf.

International Safe Harbor Privacy Principles, http://www.trade.gov/td/ecom/shprin.html (accessed May 23, 2010).

Jane E. Brody, "Medical Paper Trail Takes Electronic Turn," *New York Times*, February 22, 2010, http://www.nytimes.com/2010/02/23/health/23brod.html.

Jesse C. Vivian, "Pharmacists Beware: Data Mining Unlawful," U.S.Pharmacist.com, June 18, 2009, http://www.uspharmacist.com/content/d/pharmacy_law/c/13856/.

Jilian Mincer, "Patient ID Theft Rises," *Wall Street Journal* Online, November 29, 2009, http://online.wsj.com/article/SB125944755514168145.html.

Joe Killian, "Stolen Laptop has Information on 14,000 Moses Cane Patients," *News & Record*, April 14, 2009, http://www.news-record.com/content/2009/04/13/article/laptop_stolen_contains_information_from_14000_moses_cone_patients.

Karen Singer, "ObamaCare: This Might Hurt," Conntact.com, May 10, 2010, http://www.conntact.com/health/10367-obamacare-this-might-hurt.html.

Katherine Capps and John B. Harkey, "Employee Health and Productivity Programs: The Use of Incentives," June 2008, http://www.incentone.com/files/2008-surveyresults.pdf.

The Kaiser Foundation and Health Research Education Trust, "Employee Health Benefits, 2008 Annual Survey," http://ehbs.kff.org/pdf/7790.pdf.

Kevin Kwang, "Job Hunters Should Avoid Risky Online Behavior," ZDNet Asia, May 7, 2010, http://www.zdnetasia.com/job-hunters-should-avoid-risky-online-behavior-62063098.htm.

Kim Zetter, "New Law Floods California With Medical Data Breach Reports," *Wired*, July 9, 2009, http://www.wired.com/threatlevel/2009/07/health-breaches/#ixzz0fc9ffk6r.

"Laptop with Patient Info Stolen," *Rocky Mountain News*, November 29, 2006, http://m.rockymountainnews.com/news/2006/Nov/29/laptop-with-patient-info-stolen/.

Lisa Wangsness, "Electronic Health Records Raise Doubt," *Boston Globe*, April 13, 2009, http://www.boston.com/news/nation/washington/articles/2009/04/13/electronic_health_records_raise_doubt/.

Liz Freeman, "Florida Health Fraud Case Breaks New Legal Ground," *Naples Daily News*, September 15, 2006, http://www.naplesnews.com/news/2006/sep/15/florida_health_fraud_case_breaks_new_legal_ground/?local_news.

Lisa Girion and Ricardo Alonso, "Steep Rise Projected for Health Spending," *L.A. Times*, February 22, 2006, http://articles.latimes.com/2006/feb/22/business/fi-healthcost22.

Luca Mearian, "Health Net Says 1.5M Medical Records Lost in Data Breach: Connecticut A.G. Calls Six-Month Delay in Reporting Loss 'Incomprehensible,'" *Computer World*, November 19, 2009, http://www.computerworld.com/s/article/9141172/Health_Net_says_1.5M_medical_records_lost_in_data_breach.

"Medical Records Confidentiality: Issues Affecting the Mental Health and Substance Abuse Systems," posting of John Petrila, petrila@mirage.fmhi.usf.edu, to Med-Privacy@essential.org, April 28, 1999.

MedicAlert, http://www.medicalert.org/.

Melissa Weddle and Patricia K. Kokotailo, "Confidentiality and Consent in Adolescent Substance Abuse: An Update," *AMA J. Ethics,* March 2005, http://virtualmentor.ama-assn.org/2005/03/pfor1-0503.html.

"Mental Health: A Report of the Surgeon General, Chapter 7 Current State of Confidentiality Law," http://www.surgeongeneral.gov/library/mentalhealth/chapter7/sec3.html.

Michelle Andrews, "Medical Identity Theft Turns Patients Into Victims," *U.S. News and World Report*, February 29, 2008, http://www.usnews.com/health/family-health/articles/2008/02/29/medical-identity-theft-turns-patients-into-victims.html.

Michael Savage, "NHS 'Loses' Thousands of Medical Records," *The Independent*, May 25, 2009, http://www.independent.co.uk/news/uk/politics/nhs-loses-thousands-of-medical-records-1690398.html.

Microsoft HealthVault and HIPAA, June 2009, http://msdn.microsoft.com/en-us/healthvault/cc507320.aspx (accessed April 9, 2010).

Milt Freudenheim, "And You Thought a Prescription Was Private," *New York Times*, August 8, 2009, http://www.nytimes.com/2009/08/09/business/09privacy.html?sq=de-identified%20health%20data&st=cse&scp=1&pagewanted=all.

Miriam Wugmeister and Nathan D. Taylor, "United States: Six States Now Require Social Security Number Protection Policies," Mondaq, December 10, 2008, http://www.mondaq.com/article.asp?articleid=71322.

Natasha Singer, "When 2+2 Equals a Privacy Question," *New York Times*, October 17, 2009, http://www.nytimes.com/2009/10/18/business/18stream.html?scp=3&sq=%22de-identified%22&st=cse.

New York State Office of Mental Health, "New York State Office of Mental Health HIPAA Prempetion Analysis," http://www.omh.state.ny.us/omhweb/hipaa/preemption_html/MHLARTICLE31-33-43.htm#3313.

"N.W.T. Medical Records Faxed to CBC," CBC.com, May 11, 2010, http://www.cbc.ca/canada/north/story/2010/05/11/nwt-medical-records-fax.html

"N.Y. Hospital Employee Admits Stealing, Selling Patient Data," *Campus Safety*, April 14, 2008, http://www.campussafetymagazine.com/News/?NewsID=1851.

Office for Civil Rights, "HIPAA Compliance and Enforcement," 2008, http://www.hhs.gov/ocr/privacy/enforcement/.

Office of the Privacy Commissioner (Australia), "Privacy in the Private Health Sector," November 9, 2001, http://www.privacy.gov.au/materials/types/guidelines/view/6517 (accessed April 14, 2010).

Office of the Privacy Commissioner of Canada, "Legal Information Related to PIPEDA: Interpretations (Personal Information)," http://www.priv.gc.ca/leg_c/interpretations_02_e.cfm (accessed May 17, 2010).

Office of the Privacy Commissioner of Canada, "Summaries of Cases Settled During the Course of the Investigation Under the Personal Information Protection and Electronic Documents Act, http://www.privcom.gc.ca/ser/index_01_e.asp (accessed April 14, 2010).

Office of the Privacy Commissioner of Canada, "Summary of an Early Resolution Case Under the Personal Information Protection and Electronic Documents Act," http://www.privcom.gc.ca/ser/index_02_e.asp (accessed April 14, 2010).

Office of the Privacy Commissioner of Canada, "Your Privacy Responsibilities: Canada's Personal Information Protection and Electronic Documents Act," http://www.priv.gc.ca/information/guide_e.pdf (accessed May 17, 2010).

Organization of Economic Co-operation & Development, "OECD Guidelines on the Protection of Privacy and Transborder Flows of Personal Data," September 23, 1980 http://www.oecd.org/document/18/0,2340,en_2649 _34255_1815186_1_1_1_1,00.html.

PatientPrivacyRights.org, "UPI Poll: Concern on Health Privacy (2007)," http://www.patientprivacyrights.org/site/News2?page=NewsArticle&id=6796&news_iv_ctrl=1241.

"Physicians File Lawsuit on FTC's Red Flags Rule," American Medical Association Online, May 21, 2010, http://www.ama-assn.org/ama/pub/news/news/lawsuit-red-flags-rule.shtml.

The Prescription Project, "Fact Sheet: Prescription Data Mining," November 19, 2008, http://www.prescriptionproject.org/tools/initiatives_factsheets/files/0004.pdf.

Privacy Act of 1988 (Australia), http://www.comlaw.gov.au/ComLaw/Legislation/ActCompilation1.nsf/framelodgmentattachments/80B97C0EECC31CA4CA25 76BF007FBEBD (accessed April 14, 2010).

Questions presented on May 4, 2006, by the ABA Joint Committee on Employee Benefits, http://www.abanet.org/jceb/2006/EEOC2006final.pdf.

Rebecca C. Jones, *Living With HIV/AIDS: Students Tell Their Stories of Stigma, Courage, and Resillience* 22–32 (2006), http://www.nsba.org/MainMenu/SchoolHealth/SelectedNSBAPublications/HIVAIDS.aspx.

Records, Computers and the Rights of Citizens: Report of the Secretary's Advisory Committee on Automated Personal Data Systems, http://aspe.hhs.gov/datacncl/1973privacy/c3.htm.

Robert Mackey, "Depressed Woman Appears Happy on Facebook, Trouble Ensues," *New York Times* News Blog, November 23, 2009, http://thelede.blogs.nytimes.com/2009/11/23/depressed-woman-appears-happy-on-facebook-trouble-ensues/?scp=1&sq=nathalie%20blanchard&st=cse.

Robin Finn, "Arthur Ashe, Tennis Star, Is Dead at 49," *New York Times*, February 8, 1993, http://www.nytimes.com/learning/general/onthisday/bday/0710.html?scp=1&sq=Arthur%20Ashe%20hospital&st=cse.

Robin A. Johnson, "The HIPAA Security Rule: CMS' Enforcement Activities Acquire Teeth," http://www.carf.org/consumer.aspx?content=content/About/Partners/SecurityRule.htm.

Roe v. Social Security Administration (03-CIV-3812; settled 2004), "The Legal Action Centers Leading Cases," http://www.lac.org/doc_library/lac/publications/leading_cases.pdf (accessed May 24, 2010).

Rosemarie Bernardo, "Woman Who Revealed AIDS Info Gets a Year," *Honolulu Star Bulletin*, June 10, 2009, http://www.starbulletin.com/news/20090610_Woman_who_revealed_AIDS_info_gets_a_year.html.

Sarah C. Swider and Mark C. Suchman, "Taking Notice: Public Perceptions of Health Privacy in the Wake of HIPAA," paper presented at the annual meeting of the American Sociological Association, New York, August 11, 2007, http://www.allacademic.com//meta/p_mla_apa_research_citation/1/8/5/1/1/pages185111/p185111-5.php.

Sid Kirchheimer, "Scam Alert: Stealing Your Health by Medical Identity Theft," *AARP Bulletin Today*, September 2006, http://bulletin.aarp.org/yourmoney/scamalert/articles/scam_alert__stealing.html.

"State Profile: Nydia M. Velazquez," *USA Today* Online, http://content.usatoday.com/news/politicselections/CandidateProfile.aspx?ci=1535&oi=H (accessed March 26, 2010).

Stephanie Couelgnoux, "Laptop Stolen From Halifax Health Employee's Car," *Central Florida News* 13, October 15, 2009, http://www.cfnews13.com/News/Local/2009/10/14/laptop_stolen_from_halifax_health_employees_car.html.

Steven Greenhouse and Martin Barbaro, *New York Times*, October 26, 2005,,http://www.nytimes.com/2005/10/26/Business/26walmart.ready.html?pagewanted=1&_r=1.

U.S. Department of Health & Human Services, "Frequently Asked Questions About the Disposal of Protected Health Information," http://www.hhs.gov/ocr/privacy/hipaa/enforcement/examples/disposalfaqs.pdf (accessed February 28, 2010).

U.S. Department of Health & Human Services, "HHS, Providence Health Agree on Corrective Action Plan to Protect Health Information," http://www.hhs.gov/ocr/privacy/hipaa/enforcement/examples/providenceresolutionagreement.html.

Walecia Konrad, "Medical Problems Could Include Identity Theft," *New York Times*, June 12, 2009, http://www.nytimes.com/2009/06/13/health/13patient.html?_r=1.

Wendy Davis, "Court: Posting Medical Info On MySpace Violates Privacy," MediaPost, June 28, 2009, http://www.mediapost.com/publications/index.cfm?fa=Articles.showArticle&art_aid=108791.

"Working Document on the Processing of Personal Data Relating to Health in Electronic Health Records," http://ec.europa.eu/justice_home/fsj/privacy/docs/wpdocs/2007/wp131_en.pdf (accessed May 23, 2010).

Appendicies

Appendix A: Consumer Checklist for Responding to Medical Identity Theft

Recommended Action	Resources	Date/Notes
Obtain copies of credit reports; review reports; make corrections where needed and place fraud alerts on file.	All Americans are entitled to a free credit report every year from each of the three major credit bureaus as a result of the passage of the 2003 Fair and Accurate Credit Transactions Act. Online: Go to http://www.annualcreditreport.com. This is the only authorized source for consumers to access their annual credit report online for free. Phone: You can also call 1-877-322-8228. Mail: You may complete the form on the back of the Annual Credit Report Request brochure, and mail it to Annual Credit Report Request Service, P.O. Box 105281, Atlanta, GA, 30348-5281. The brochure is available at https://www.annualcreditreport.com/cra /requestformfinal.pdf, and all three credit reports may be requested at one time.	
Request an accounting of disclosures from covered entities.	Use your provider's form, or if the provider does not have its own form, consider using the sample provided in this book or another similar form.	

(*Continued*)

Recommended Action	Resources	Date/Notes
If a Social Security number has been compromised or is suspected of being used inappropriately, contact the Social Security Administration's fraud hotline.	Social Security Administration Fraud Reporting 1-800-269-0271 http://www.ssa.gov/oig/guidelin.htm	
Review FTC resources, including the Tool for Victims.	FTC Tool for Victims: http://www.ftc.gov/bcp/edu/microsites/idtheft/tools.html	
Consider completing the universal affidavit form and providing completed copies of it to all creditors	See the FTC universal affidavit form and follow directions for completing the same: http://www.ftc.gov/bcp/edu/resources/forms/affidavit.pdf	
Request copies of health records and review for any inaccuracies. Make sure all inaccuracies have been corrected prior to seeking health care.	Use the forms provided by the applicable health care provider or insurer, or if none are available, use the sample forms for requesting access to medical records in Chapter 2.	
Notify your health care providers and health plans promptly in the event of any identified fraud.	Contact the health information manager or the privacy officer at the provider organization or the antifraud hotline at the health plan where the medical identity theft appears to have occurred.	

File a police report and send copies with correct information to insurers, providers, and credit bureaus once the identity theft has been confirmed.	Contact your local police station.
Take detailed notes of all conversations related to the medical identity theft. Write down the date, name, and contact information of everyone contacted, as well as the content of the conversation.	Maintain the notes in a secure place.
Make copies of any letters, reports, documents, and e-mail sent or received regarding the identity theft.	Maintain the copies in a secure place.
Consider filing a complaint with the Identity Theft Data Clearinghouse, operated by the Federal Trade Commission and the Internet Crime Complaint Center.	Information available for filing a complaint can be found at https://rn.ftc.gov/pls/dod/widtpubl$.startup?Z_ORG_CODE=PU03
File a complaint with the attorney general in the state where the identity theft occurred.	The National Association of Attorneys General provides state-by-state information at http://www.naag.org/attorneys_general.php.

(Continued)

Recommended Action	Resources	Date/Notes
In the case of stolen or misdirected mail, contact the U.S. Postal Service.	Contact the U.S. Postal Service at 1-800-275-8777 to obtain the number of the local U.S. postal inspector.	Also see http://usps.whitepages.com/post_office.
Telecheck: 1-800-366-2425 http://www.telecheck.com	Check Services Company: 1-800-526-5380 http://www.internationalservicecheck.com/en	If a thief has stolen checks, contact your bank as well as check verification companies Telecheck and International Service Check to place a fraud alert on the account to ensure that counterfeit checks will be refused.
	Check with state authorities for resources. Many states provide consumer protection and education related to insurance and accept online complaints.	To determine if a state has a state insurance department for online complaints, visit the National Association of Insurance Commissioners at http://www.naic.org and file a complaint as appropriate.
	Work with the organization where the medical identity theft occurred to stop the flow of the incorrect information, correct the existing inaccurate health record entries, and determine where incorrect information was sent.	It may not always be possible to track down the origins of the identity theft. However, when you can, it will often be helpful to work closely with the organization where it all started to eradicate the effects of the theft.
	In the event of suspected Medicare or Medicaid fraud, contact the Department of Health and Human Services.	Department of Health and Human Services 1-800-368-1019 http://www.hhs.gov/ocr

Appendix B: Additional Web Resources for Further Information

Topic or Issues	Resource and URL
Comprehensive Medical Privacy Resources	The Health Privacy Project http://www.healthprivacy.org
	World Privacy Forum http://www.worldprivacyforum.org
	Electronic Privacy Information Center (EPIC) http://epic.org/privacy/medical/
	American Civil Liberties Union (ACLU) http://www.aclu.org/ technology-and-liberty/ medical-privacy
	Privacilla Resources on Medical Privacy http://www.privacilla.org/medical.html
	Pew Internet Resources on Health http:// www.pewinternet.org/topics/Health.aspx
Employee Background Checks and Health Privacy	Privacy Rights Clearinghouse http://www .privacyrights.org/fs/fs16-bck.htm
	FTC Resource http://www.ftc.gov/bcp/ edu/pubs/business/credit/bus08.shtm
Health IT Issues	Connecting for Health (Markle Foundation) http://www.connectingforhealth.org/
Insurance Issues	FTC Guide for Insurers http://www.ftc .gov/bcp/edu/pubs/business/credit/ bus07.shtm
State-Specific Guides on Accessing Your Medical Records	Georgetown University, Center on Medical Records Rights and Privacy http://medicalrecordrights.georgetown .edu/records.html
Listing of State Attorneys General	National Association of Attorneys General http://www.naag.org/current- attorneys-general.php
AMA Resources on Patient Confidentiality	American Medical Association http://www .ama-assn.org/ama/pub/ physician-resources/legal-topics/ patient-physician-relationship-topics/ patient-confidentiality.shtml

Appendix C: Key Privacy Agencies by Jurisdiction

Jurisdiction	Web Site
Argentina: National Directorate for Personal Data Protection	http://www.jus.gov.ar/
Australia: Office of the Privacy Commissioner	http://www.privacy.gov.au
Austria: Austrian Data Protection Commission	http://www.dsk.gv.at
Belgium: Commission for the Protection of Privacy	http://www.privacycommission.be
Canada: Office of the Privacy Commissioner	http://www.priv.gc.ca
Cyprus: Office for the Commission of Personal Data Protection	http://www.dataprotection.gov.cy
Czech Republic: Office for Personal Data Protection	http://www.uoou.cz
Denmark: Data Protection Agency	http://www.datatilsynet.dk/english/
France: CNIL	http://www.cnil.fr
Germany: Federal Commissioner for Data Protection and Freedom of Information	http://www.bfdi.bund.de
Greece: Hellenic Data Protection Authority	http://www.dpa.gr
Hungary: Hungarian Parliamentary Commissioner for Data Protection and Freedom of Information	http://abiweb.obh.hu/dpc/
Iceland: Data Protection Authority	http://www.personuvernd.is
Ireland: Data Protection Commissioner	http://www.dataprotection.ie/
Italy: Data Protection Commissioner	http://www.garanteprivacy.it
Luxembourg: National Commission for Data Protection	http://www.cnpd.public.lu
Netherlands: Dutch Data Protection Authority	http://www.dutchdpa.nl
New Zealand: Privacy Commissioner	http://www.privacy.org.nz

Norway: Data Inspectorate http://www.datatilsynet.no

Poland: Inspector General for Personal Data Protection http://www.giodo.gov.pl

Portugal: National Commission of Data Protection http://www.cnpd.pt

Romania: National Commission for Personal Data Processing http://www.dataprotection.ro

Slovakia: Office for Personal Data Protection http://www.ico.gov.uk

Slovenia: Data Protection Authority http://www.ip-rs.si

Spain: Spanish Data Protection Agency http://www.agpd.es

Sweden: Swedish Data Inspection Board http://www.datainspektionen.se

Switzerland: Federal Data Protection and Information Commissioner http://www.edoeb.admin.ch

United Kingdom: Information Commissioner's Office http://www.ico.gov.uk

United States: California Office of Privacy Protection http://www.privacy.ca.gov

United States: Department of Health and Human Services http://www.hhs.gov

United States: Federal Trade Commission http://www.ftc.gov

Index

ABOUT THE AUTHOR

Jacqueline Klosek, a certified information privacy professional, is an attorney in private practice with Goodwin Procter LLP in New York, where she focuses on advising clients on issues related to data privacy and security and negotiating various technology agreements. She is the author of *The Right to Know: Your Guide to Using and Defending Freedom of Information Law in the United States* (Praeger, 2009), *The War on Privacy* (Praeger, 2006), *The Legal Guide to E-Business* (Greenwood Publishing, 2003), and *Data Privacy in the Information Age* (Greenwood Publishing, 2000). She is completing a manuscript for her sixth book, to be titled, *Why Healthcare Reform is Not Enough* (Potomac Books, 2011). She is a coauthor of the third edition of *Cyberlaw: Text and Cases* (Cengage, 2010). Klosek received *NJBiz* magazine's 40 Under 40 award, given annually to the top 40 achievers in New Jersey with an established record of leadership who have taken on key decision-making roles at an earlier-than-usual stage in their lives. She was also the recipient of the Telford-Taylor Fellowship in Public International Law. She is a graduate of the Vrije Universiteit in Brussels (LLM, European and international law), the Benjamin N. Cardozo School of Law (JD, law), and New York University (BA, psychology). She is a board member of the Internet Bar Organization. She has her own radio program called "Your Right to Health," which airs on HealthBeat Radio, a health channel powered by Lucy Radio Networks LLC. She may be reached for comment through her Web site at http://www .jacquelineklosek.com.